BE STILL AND KNOW I'M

GOD

PSALM 46:10

A Caregiver's Journey through Parents' Alzheimer's and Dementia

Teresa Williams Trotter

ISBN 978-1-63630-664-3 (Paperback)
ISBN 978-1-63630-665-0 (Digital)

Cover photo: *The resting place of Benny and Grace, along the shore of their lake.*

Covenant Books, Inc.
11661 Hwy 707
Murrells Inlet, SC 29576
www.covenantbooks.com

What people are saying…

"With humor, humility and honesty, Teresa Trotter shares her moving journey of caring for her beloved parents as she watches them mentally and physically slip away from her. Finding herself in the role of caregiver to the people who nurtured her throughout her life is a jarring and sometimes quite painful experience. But with the support of her family, friends and her faith, she confronts the myriad of responsibilities and feelings of helplessness with grace and gratitude. As she faces the logistical and emotional tasks of saying goodbye, she finds the power of love and precious memories prevail. For anyone who is facing similar challenges in caring for an ailing loved one—or even those who are not—Teresa's story is a compelling read that is well worth the time."

—Trevis Mayfield,
President, Sycamore Media,
Maquoketa Sentinel-Press, Bellevue Herald-Leader,
DeWitt Observer, Eastern Iowa Farmer

"Grab a comfortable chair and a box of Kleenex and get ready to laugh and cry. You will get totally caught up in Teresa's raw and brutally honest retelling of her experiences dealing with first her father's and then also her mother's (at the same time) health decline into the world of Alzheimer's disease. Not only will you hear some of the family history, influential characters and intriguing adventures, but also the world-altering impact the disease had on all. Teresa bares her soul as she reveals all of the emotions, good and bad, that overcame her during the difficult journey. She also generously shares practical advice she gained when dealing with challenges arising from choices that had to be made for the care of her diseased loved ones.

This is a great read for anyone whose friend or family member is beginning to show the signs of dementia. You will be comforted as well as enlightened. You will know that God has stood by others facing what you now face and carried them to the other side. Learn how Teresa benefitted by making time to *Be Still and Know I'm God* carried her through the most difficult time in her life. You'll be truly blessed!"

—Linda Hood,
natural health coach, Naturopath, CNHP (Certified Natural Health Professional), CECP (Certified Emotion Code Practitioner), CPT (Certified Personal Trainer)

"It is in the moment that we release our grip and be still before God that His work through our lives breathes loudest. God works all things together for good when we fully depend on Him. In Teresa's transparent, fearless journey in battling the attempt by Alzheimer's disease to demolish her parent's life, God showed up in a pervasive way to bring triumph. This is a must read for anyone who feels they are facing debilitating disease alone. It is a guide to make wise decisions and lean on the presence of God in the lives of those He brings into your life to win the daily battles. You will be victorious when you *Be Still and Know He is God*!"

—Keith Smith, Minister of Dade Christian Church

"Have you lost a parent or perhaps a loved one to a disease related to aging? A Caregiver's Journey is a tender, honest and beautifully written memoir that explores the emotional journey of caring for aging parents diagnosed with Alzheimer's disease and dementia. Being someone who has lost both parents, I identified with the emotional word pictures presented. Precious conversations and memories are shared in an intimate story that invites you to know the author in a deep and meaningful way. We will be blessed through the storms of our lives when we remain still and know that God is in control."

—Jennifer Smith,
teacher and professional storyteller,
mother of four children, in ministry with
her husband for thirty years

"*Alzheimer's. Dementia.* Those words tend to frighten, isolate and anger. Teresa Trotter takes us through a daughter's journey into a world we hope we never have to see. She gives great insight into the life of the caregiver.

"Her brutal honesty about how she did not handle certain situations well is a great encouragement to those that think they have to have all the answers.

"Caregivers will find great comfort and guidance from Teresa's experiences. Talking to siblings can be tricky, but Teresa discusses how she approached her family members.

"Teresa Trotter exposes her deepest emotions, fears and hopes in this book. Her raw emotions let the reader know that they are not alone in their feelings. Caregivers think they have to be superhuman. In the way that only Teresa can, she makes it clear that no one is superhuman, and all need God to sustain them in the darkest times.

"If you have found yourself being the caregiver of an elder and aren't ready to talk to anyone yet, please read this book. You will feel like you have found a friend and kindred spirit in Teresa Trotter."

—Beth Clark, residential care administrator

"In this autobiographical narrative, Teresa Williams Trotter authentically shares her experience as a caregiver for her parents suffering from dementia. She tells how the inspirational love story they had been living shifted to days of confusion and danger for her mother and daddy. Trotter honestly describes feelings of helplessness, anger, fear and sadness. Her words of raw vulnerability are a true gift to the caregiving community, allowing others to know they are not alone in this overwhelming, intimate space. She balances intense feelings with ultimate strength in her faith and gratitude for those who've companioned her on this journey.

"Readers will connect with the detailed emotional changes throughout the course of witnessing transitions in the identities of her mother and father. Trotter writes with a descriptive voice that made me feel like I was once again sitting next to her in a rocking chair on the front porch, hearing stories of the beautiful way her parents loved one another and the fun life they shared! Just like many years ago, I could envision them side by side in an old, restored carriage, taking a leisurely drive around the family-owned property. Though this book is an account of her individual experience, the battles with anticipatory grief and navigating self-care while balancing everyday life will be relevant to all children who find themselves in these caregiver shoes."

—Rev. Allissa Santoro Williams,
MDiv, MAMHC, CCTP, CNA, CDP, regional spirituality director and mental health counselor

CONTENTS

FOREWORD

When I began writing this story four years ago, I thought its purpose would primarily be to help me release all the grief, pain and frustration of dealing with the preceding years of caring for my parents. I felt it would perhaps be a cleansing of my soul to get all these thoughts on paper, where I could put them into perspective.

Why did it take four years to write? Because sometimes the pain would be so overwhelming, I would simply have to stop for a while. My feelings were still too raw. I would cry and leave it alone for weeks or months. Then the drive to tell this story would come back, and I would write until the flood of emotion swept over me again.

During this process, I came to realize that this is not just *my* story. It is the story of anyone who has ever been in this situation, of caring for aging parents. Then it dawned on me that it is also for anyone who has ever served as a caregiver for someone with any debilitating disease—cancer, Lou Gehrig's, Parkinson's, you name it.

Within my story are nuggets of truth that other caregivers may find immensely helpful so that they do not have to reinvent the wheel. Some of the approaches we took to my parents' care can be applied in any situation, like keeping a daily care journal or adding all the holistic and detailed features we included in their care. The steps we took to renovate their home to enhance their care may even give helpful tips to other caregivers.

Beyond that, I was struck by how alone I felt during this ordeal, and yet thousands of others have gone through similar situations. Perhaps just knowing that you are not alone, nor are you the first to deal with such a storm of emotions, might help *you*, as a caregiver, in your own journey.

My deepest thanks to my family and friends for supporting and encouraging me in this endeavor. But most of all, I thank the Lord for giving me the strength to endure revisiting the painful moments and for helping me find the joy and release in celebrating my parents' lives.

I am thankful that He helped me to be still and know that He is, indeed, God.

CHAPTER 1

In the Beginning

It is a beautiful evening. I feel the wind in my face and the comfort of a restored vintage "Big Red" 1976 Cadillac Eldorado convertible. The word *pristine* doesn't even touch it. It is in a class out of this world. This car was one of those big sleek cars that in a parade carried the queen. That evening, I felt like riding on the back, waving like a queen. The queen of peace, my peace. My mind went back to that year, 1976, when I was two years out of high school, in college, and married with a one-year-old little girl. Everyone was younger and healthy. Somehow, I never thought about where I would be and what I would be doing forty-one years later.

I do know a couple of things that I have learned over the years. Life is never to be taken for granted because you truly do not know from minute to minute what could happen. *Love*, I know that is a big word, but love family and friends around you. Life is short.

The couple who owns this car are our best friends. The fun, the talks and friendship that we have shared over the years are one of a kind. I believe the toughest of times we have shared have been the passing of parents. Dennis, Sharon and I shared the passing of our parents within months apart. The help we gave each

> **"I did come out stronger, but not without hurt and bruising on this journey."**

other was monumental. Sometimes it was just being there, not saying a word, and sometimes listening to incredibly sad situations. It helped knowing we each shared the same emotions.

Thoughts of yesterday rush through my mind. Those thoughts that I have are warm thoughts and steadfast. It has taken me awhile to get to this place in my heart. It hasn't been without a battle, without coping with depression, without anger. It has been a climb out of the bottom of a hole that was the size of Montana. I thank God daily, I thank family, I thank friends. Without those three, life would be nothing.

What a beautiful evening. What a wonderful ride. Thank you, Daddy and Mother, for giving me life. It is hard for me to believe I made it through to this point, cruising down the state highway. My heart shattered many times in the last five years, and I would not have believed I would have this smile on my face ever again.

I did come out stronger, but not without hurt and bruising on this journey, and it has been a long one. My personal growth has been immeasurable. I do not proclaim that I know everything about that ugly disease Alzheimer's, but I do know the only way through this disease is one day at a time, and God will carry you through. Love for God, love for family, love for friends are the most important values in life. I genuinely believe you cannot make it through without those. Here is my story.

CHAPTER 2

Psalm 46:10

Be still, and know that I am God; I will be exalted among the nations, I will be exalted in the earth.

God states, "Be still and know I'm God." So many times, on my journey with caregiving for my parents, I had so many emotions run through me. At times I wanted to get in a fetal position and stay there, but knowing I had work to do and caregiving, that was not possible. I felt the pain of letting go of a time when all was well. I watched them become strangers before my eyes. Just pieces of them were recognizable. Other times I felt as if I were alien to my surroundings.

The hurt of Alzheimer's disease is brutal for the one that has been diagnosed with the disease and for the family watching the disease destroy their family member. It is a disease that, at times, takes years to destroy a person. They go from life, full of energy, happiness and joy to confusion to eventually not knowing who they are or not being able to recognize their loved ones around them.

I cannot watch the movie *The Notebook* and not think of my mother and daddy. In that movie, the female lead develops dementia, just like my mother did. I honestly think the love story in that film has many similarities to my parents' lives. Daddy came home from World War II, and he and Mother fell in love. They married in 1947. They raised three children, celebrating the birth of their first child,

Janet, in 1947, James in 1950, myself in 1956. They built a successful business starting in 1960 and sold it in 1980. Daddy retired at the age of fifty-five. They bought a beautiful 130-acre farm in southern Vigo County in Indiana in 1966. After Daddy retired from the veterinary supply business, he spent many days on the farm caring for the horses and cattle.

Daddy enjoyed his farm, and he kept it looking like a park. Mother told of Daddy's diagnosis of Alzheimer's disease in 2009. I suspect the diagnosis was actually a few years before that. We had gone to Hawaii in 2003

> "I felt the pain of letting go of a time when all was well."

together, and he had some memory problems, nothing serious. As you look back, you just wonder and question what all you missed seeing.

It seems to me that both my parents' lives and the plot of the movie have the same outcome. The person with AD can no longer recognize themselves, loved ones or friends.

Dementia is a chronic and persistent disorder of the mental processes caused by brain disease or injury and by memory disorders, personality changes and impaired reasoning, leading to mental illness, madness, insanity, derangement, lunacy.

Alzheimer's disease is a progressive mental deterioration that can occur in middle or old age due to generalized degeneration of the brain. It is the most common cause of premature senility. It is a degenerative brain disease of unknown cause that is the most common form of dementia. It results in progressive memory loss, impaired thinking, disorientation and changes in personality and mood, and that is all marked histologically by the degeneration of the brain.

To me, there are so many similarities that I'm not sure why they are called by different names. I know the experts have it all lined out and can tell you practically cell by cell the difference. I experienced it with both parents, and it is heartbreaking. It doesn't matter which name you call it. I'm not a doctor, but I do know from firsthand experience that the outcome is unimaginable. I had trouble every single day comprehending why, why, why this was happening to two people who were so full of life.

The emotional journey is one that I compare to a roller coaster ride, up and down with turns and twists. The Screaming Eagle at a local theme park has nothing on this one. There are days you feel beat up, hurt, drained of your energy. You feel at times that you are sliding down a dark tunnel and you have no idea what will be at the end. There are times you pray it will end and then feel extremely guilty for that prayer.

Every time I felt myself getting out of control, a calm voice would repeat the words "Be still and know I'm God." The search for the right words, the right actions, the right care ended with me knowing that God was there, and He was in control.

"Be still and know I'm God." *I'm God.*

CHAPTER 3

My Husband, My Hero

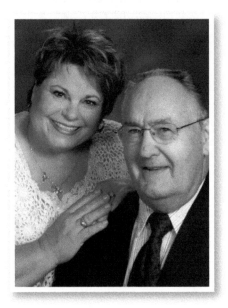

I'm sure my husband was quite curious through this book-writing process of mine. When I have mentioned various people throughout this book as being towers of strength and support, he has probably thought, *Wow! They didn't live with you.* I'm sure all women that are married to wonderful men say they are wonderful.

I have tried to collect my thoughts about a man that I have known for many years. By no means is he perfect. Sometimes he can say something that makes sense to him, that he thinks is reasonable, but when those words come out of his mouth, it isn't exactly what a woman wants to hear. I have learned over the years that men do think entirely differently from women, and sometimes that is perfect.

How is this manifested? Sometimes all the touchy-feely platitudes need to be out of the conversation. Sometimes you don't need reassuring words that begin to sound like mere platitudes. You just need plain truth. You need a rock to lean on to keep you from falling off the cliff.

During this journey that I have been on for the last several years, I wouldn't have wanted to be with anyone else. He has been my rock, my support, my light in the darkness. He always knew how to calm the storms. He was my bootstraps and my boots when I couldn't even find my boots. He has been my mind; he has helped me through tough times and has been with me in good times. He has shared my memories and held the tissues for me to blow my nose. He didn't react when I was so mad and angry, when I vented and ranted and had tantrums like a five-year-old.

He loved me through every minute. There were times I felt out of my mind with wanting to fix the problems, cure the illness, rewind to better and happier times. He was patient with me through every step of the heartbreak. He gave me space—that was a hard one—because being a woman, I wanted space, and then I was upset because it was too much space. I'm sure there were times he felt like shooting me because he was so exasperated with me. I have no doubt in my mind he was often confused and upset with me. At times, he may have felt like *he* was losing it.

Through it all, he was my husband, my supporter, my comforter. He spoke words of wisdom; he had excellent judgment. He is an individual who is sound in his decisions. I could not have made it through without him. I just pray that he has forgiven me for times of craziness. I'm sure we have many more journeys ahead of us.

This is a second marriage for both of us. We have five adult children together. We have four beautiful daughters: Nicol, Shanon, Annette and Amanda. Two of the four daughters have given us seven grandchildren, and our one son, Blaine, and his wife, Emely, have given us five grandchildren. Yes, that is twelve grandchildren total, and one of those grandchildren (Ryan) has given us one great-grandchild. Yes, we are very blessed. Our families have blended well.

However, I will reiterate that we have many journeys ahead. We will face our own aging, health issues, our retirement years, watching our grandchildren make difficult decisions. The list is lengthy. One thing I can count on, through it all, we will carry each other. Where one is weak, the other one will carry. Being strong for one another is what a true marriage is all about.

CHAPTER 4

Drive Off Sunday

When my husband, Joe, and I married, it was a second marriage for us both. Joe's parents had died many years before. Joe told me when we got married, "Enjoy your parents, Teresa, because they will not be with us forever." How right he was. I wish there had been more Sundays and special occasions to be together. I miss those times so much.

Joe loved my mother and daddy. They loved to play cards and enjoyed being at our home on Sundays for dinner and the kids all coming home. Mother would call when they got home and say, "We had such a good time! Thanks for having us."

Easter Sunday 2011 was the worst day imaginable. The stress and the emotions of that day were chilling. It was a day that I will never forget. The uncertainty of how that day would end was just about more than a human could handle or what I thought I could handle. Mother and Daddy were coming to our house as always for Easter dinner and the Easter egg hunt with all their great-grandkids.

I was busy preparing the meal and all the last-minute things you do getting ready for company. As always, twelve noon was the appointed time, and Mother and Daddy would always arrive about thirty minutes early—never, never late. Eleven thirty came, no parents. Noon came, no parents. At 12:05 p.m., I was on the phone.

Mother answered, and she said Daddy had gone down to the end of the lane to the mailbox to get her Sunday paper about 7:45 a.m., and he never came back.

I was stunned, and I started to panic. I was trying to stay calm. I asked, "Mother, have you called the police?"

"Yes," she said. "A few minutes ago. They just got here."

I have to say that at that point, I was confused as to my mother's lack of concern and waiting four hours to call the police. In my heart, in my mind, I was just about two seconds away from losing control. This is where your mind runs away with you.

Let me explain. Have you ever gone through the house of horrors at the county fair? You are running through mazes, trying to find your way out, and each way you choose is a dead end, and you can feel yourself starting to panic. That feeling intensifies with each wrong turn you make. The panic takes hold, the scared feeling grows, then the mind is off and running.

You envision horrible things. Will he be found? If we do find him, will he be alive? Did Dad decide to drive to a strip pit somewhere and think he was going to go fishing and fall in and drown? Did some crazy person somewhere see his confused state and take advantage of an old man? Will the police find him in the trunk of the car, dead? Or in a cornfield somewhere, robbed and beaten to death? All these horrific scenarios race through your mind. Terror, fear, panic. All the questions run rampant.

> **"The stress and the emotion of that day were chilling."**

Then another thought crept into my mind. Was my father aware of his Alzheimer's disease? Did he know when he was diagnosed that this was a type of illness that takes every fabric of your being and makes it unknown to yourself? Did he understand that a person never beats this illness and never gets well? Would he take his own life? Did he see that this would not be a life he would want, not knowing himself or his loved ones around him? All those thoughts are in your mind every minute that your loved one is missing.

Frantically, places are racing through your head, and you want to be at every one of those places at the same time to see if he is there. The list of emotions was lengthy. The tears fall one after another, and the worry is massive and indescribable.

The police issued a local Silver Alert, but after I talked to them, the alert went national. I had explained to them that Mother and Daddy would often cross the river into Illinois for lunch. Daddy's picture was on TV throughout the day.

Our daughter Amanda is an amazing woman. The control she exercised was extraordinary. Where she drew her strength from, I can only imagine, but I'm sure God had something to do with it. Without Amanda there keeping everyone and everything moving, I'm not sure I could have made it through the day.

I wanted to go off somewhere alone, withdraw into the fetal position and cry. Babbling would have been my language, incoherent to anyone who would have found me, but Amanda and God held me back from going over the edge. I kept my focus, but inside I was a hot mess. Those emotions that I was feeling were so confusing to me. I had always been a strong individual, an incredibly determined person. I had gone through a few intense difficulties in my life.

I married at age eighteen to my high school sweetheart. At the age of nineteen, I had a baby with a serious eye problem. Amanda was diagnosed with an eye tumor, and removal of the right eye at three months old was necessary. During the surgery, they placed a rubber ball in the socket to develop muscle movement and stimulate facial growth. It was recommended that it stay in place for twenty-four months for complete muscle and growth stimulation. Amanda developed a staph infection at the age of twenty months, and her body rejected the rubber ball in the socket.

I do have to share that I have always felt like God speaks through people at various times in our lives. I was on the elevator at Riley Hospital and had been up for about thirty-six hours with my baby daughter. I was terribly upset, hoping her temperature would go down. She had an IV in her head. Little toddlers cannot have IVs in their arms like adults because they will not leave them alone, and they usually pull them out. There was another woman on the elevator, and I must have looked like a wreck because she proceeded to ask me if I was okay.

I said, "I'm just tired, and I have been up for a while. My baby is twenty months old and has a staph infection. She has been examined by the ophthalmology team, pediatrics team and the infectious diseases team with about ten to twelve students and doctors on each team. There's not been much sleep for me or her. She had her right eye removed at three months old. This wasn't the prosthetic that caused the infection. It was the ball preparing for the prosthetic."

She listened to me intently and had a very comforting face. She said she would keep us in her prayers and also stated that the Riley Children's Hospital was one of the best. She said it sounded like Amanda would be okay and that she was in exceptionally good care.

I asked her why she was there. She said, "I had a baby a few months ago. The doctors wanted to push my baby over to the side and let it die. I said *no*! That is my baby! The doctors informed me that he had Down syndrome, two holes in his heart and no thumbs. I told them that the holes in the heart could be fixed and the thumbs could be repaired. The doctor agreed that they could but to rest assured that Down syndrome could not be fixed."

My heart went out to this woman. After listening to this lady and her story, I knew right then that yes, maybe we had some problems, but nothing like hers, and I was very thankful. I knew our problems were going to be solved. That was my first experience with *"be still and know I'm God!"*

We made frequent trips to Riley Hospital for the first two years of Amanda's life. My college studies were put on hold. I strongly dealt with crisis after crisis that occurred throughout the years. My grandparents both passed away. I went through a divorce. My son was in the Marine Corps Special Forces with thirteen deployments to Iraq and Afghanistan, and we never knew for sure if he would return. These are a few situations that I have been through in my lifetime that required control. Through all those crises, I never felt this confused or out of control in my thinking. Now I was feeling totally out of control. I could see no way that this situation could be fixed!

I believe that seeing the changing behavior of my parents was just so foreign to me that I couldn't grasp the reality. My parents were always in control of their lives, steadfast and solid in their decision-making. They were always the ones we turned to for answers. I was having trouble coping. The feelings of how to deal with all this came out in many different thoughts, some not good but thoughts nonetheless. My mind was reeling.

Amanda is a very good organizer, a take-charge type person, and she was *on* it. With Daddy's pictures in hand, she and her team set out, asking at businesses that Mother and Daddy frequented if anyone had seen him. She was good friends with a man in the local police dispatch department, and they kept in close contact all day. There were many family members, friends and neighbors who spent the day looking for my father.

Information was being dispatched out to other local police departments in the neighboring counties. Our daughter Annette was following up by looking around the city, trying to spot the car. Everyone was trying to stay calm, but with every passing hour, the looking and praying became more frantic.

My son Blaine is a Marine, and at the time he and his family were in Virginia Beach. Blaine had just gotten back from being out of the country, and he was unable to be home with us. I called him to let him know about Grandpa driving off. Of course, he asked if he needed to come home, and I told him to just sit tight, that hopefully Grandpa would be located soon!

At that time, I worked for the Sullivan County Sheriff's Department, which is the county next to Vigo County where my parents lived. When I called my boss, Sheriff Brian Kinnett, he had his chief deputy, Dave Haddix, and another volunteer, Officer Rodriquez, look around Sullivan County for Daddy. Bryan was very serious, asking if I was okay and at the same time doing his job. He asked questions and tried to prepare me for the worst results.

I remember breaking down on the phone with him and telling him I was scared. He said it would be okay. He instructed me to try to remember Daddy's favorite fishing places, hunting places, places he had worked, the places he had lived, the places in Sullivan he liked when they came to see me. Places, places, places! It all helped, and Bryan's staff checked all those out for me. Hopefully, this situation never happens to you, but if it does, call everyone you can think of to help. Every minute is important.

My son Blaine called again in the middle of everything. In our family, sometimes the humor is a little rough, a bit wacky. Sometimes all of us will say off-the-wall stuff, and it is just plain funny. I'm not saying it is right; it is just our crazy family's way. My father loved the humor, and he could say some pretty funny things himself.

Blaine knew in his heart that I was stressing pretty badly and that it was time for funny. He said, "Mom, remember when we were kids and Grandpa hid the Easter eggs? Well, this year, Mom, he decided to hide himself!"

Blaine was laughing, and I couldn't help myself. I started crying and laughing, and for some reason at that point, I felt it was going to be okay. How, I don't know, but I just felt it would be.

All day and nothing, no news. It was starting to get dark. People checked in with me every hour, but nothing, not a trace, not a word. Throughout the day, I had hoped that Daddy was sitting somewhere, not driving around. What my boss Bryan had said to me earlier kept echoing in my head: "If he stays with the car, that is best. He'll be easier to find. However, when they get out and are wandering around, sometimes it makes it very difficult to find them."

I kept praying, "Daddy, stay with the car. Please, Daddy, just stay with the car." I don't know why daylight seems less frightening than night, but with every passing hour, night was coming upon us, and I grew more frightened. I kept praying he was safe.

We were truly fortunate that we had a lot of contacts. I felt very blessed. A lot of the people we knew personally were in law enforcement. When it started getting dark, my worry increased.

At that point, God and I had a long on-the-knees conversation. I put my faith and hope in the Lord. I was out of ideas and places. Don't get me wrong, all day my prayers had been "Please find my daddy" and "Please bring him back to us." Now my prayer was "Father, my hope and faith are in You!" Psalm 46:10 kept repeating in my mind: "Be still and know I'm God."

"I'm God," He was saying to me. "Who are you to worry?" It was as if God was telling me, "I have this. I have your back. Let me [God] do my job."

People had checked several places throughout the day to no avail. Then about 9:45 p.m. from Mount Vernon, Jefferson County, Illinois (about 160 miles from Terre Haute, Indiana), *Officer Williams* called to say they had Daddy. They had taken him to a nearby hospital there.

How stunned I was that *Officer Gary Williams* found *Benny Williams*. I had to chuckle. God answers our prayers and pleas, but He goes a step further and answers them in a way that we will know that *He is God* and *He is in charge*. *Officer Williams* found *Mr. Williams*. Nice touch, Lord.

My heart was filled with such emotion and thankfulness. A couple had found Daddy on the interstate, out of gas and wandering around beside the car. They could see that he was disoriented when he kept talking about Terre Haute, a city some distance away in another state. They gave that information to the officer they called. The officer checked his Silver Alerts, and the picture matched my dad. Officer Williams called Terre Haute, Vigo County Sheriff's Department, and then he contacted me.

My husband and I were on our way to Mount Vernon, Illinois, to pick Daddy up, PTL! I called Mom and my daughter, and of course my daughter let all the others know and posted a thank you announcement on Facebook. Family, friends and neighbors are wonderful in times of need. Our family is very blessed with a lot of awesome people who helped us throughout that nightmarish day.

We got to the hospital at about 1:00 a.m., and my dad had three nurses taking care of him, having a good time, laughing and talking to him. They knew Daddy had Alzheimer's disease, but he had a smile that would warm your heart, and he was very charming. He never met a stranger. We got him checked out and were on the road again by 2:00 a.m. What a night!

At that point, I was not worried about their car. I just wanted to get Dad home, and I just needed to know he was safe. I would either go get the car or they could ship it to us or maybe they could just crush it.

I wasn't sure at that time how that was going to go, but I really didn't care. I knew when we got home, a tough conversation was going to happen. I was not sure how I was going to tell my daddy he would not be driving again, but I would have to. I never wanted to go through another day like this one ever again.

When we got home, I didn't think it could possibly get worse, but it did. My heart broke into a million pieces. My mother did not meet us at the door. She was in the family room, not asleep but very unemotional. This told me everything. Something was seriously wrong. Her reaction was not normal, no emotion. She was almost hateful about the inconvenience. This was not my mother's normal concern about her Benny. Yes, of course, through the years they had disagreements, but you always knew they loved each other. But after sixty-four years of marriage, this was not good. I knew at that point that Mother was not thinking clearly either. It wasn't just Daddy. Houston, we have some major huge problems here.

All I wanted to do was think, cope, think, run! *Oh my*! I wanted to run! I felt sick. I needed air. I told them I would be back in the morning and that we would have to go to the doctor to find out what was going on. I said, "Dad, the doctor might tell you that you can't drive any longer."

With that, he looked like a small child and asked me why I was saying that.

I said, "Daddy, you drove off today. We had no idea where you were. We just got back from a long trip, 160 miles."

He said, "A hundred and sixty miles? You must be talking about someone else."

I said, "No, Daddy, I'm talking about what you did."

Then he said, "Someone must have taken me there."

I said, "No, Dad, you drove all that way by yourself."

He said, "If I can't drive, will Gracie be able to?"

I said, "Yes, I believe she can. We will talk more in the morning."

The sun came up, and the morning was filled with phone conversations with nurses and appointment-making. Everyone in the medical office was aware of what had happened with Daddy the day before.

I asked if the doctor could tell Daddy that he wouldn't be able to drive any longer. The nurse asked me to write a note and they would hand it to the doctor, and it would not be a problem for the doctor to recommend for him to not operate heavy equipment or vehicles. In my heart, I thought, *Thank you, God!* I was not going to be the bad guy, but this was only the beginning.

When we arrived at Mother and Daddy's house, everything was going like a usual morning. They both acted surprised to see me. I told both of them that we needed to have a conversation this morning about what had happened the day before with Daddy driving off. He had no idea what I was talking about.

The realization hit me that my mother had been covering for Daddy. I remembered back to 2009, and today it was 2011. It suddenly hit me that lots and lots of things had gone on that I knew nothing about. Once again, I felt panic. I was ashamed. I wanted to cry. I wanted to scream. *Oh my God, help me!* I prayed. *Lord God, I really need some help here!* I realized that I had stuck my head in the sand, or had I?

I knew something wasn't right, yet I kept thinking at some point Mother would say, "I can't do this anymore. Your dad is acting like this or he is doing this."

Then my soul was flooded with emotion. I felt like I was blaming her, which was not what I meant to do, but why was I finding things out like this now? Was I overreacting? Was I being too bossy? Was I asking too many questions? *Just pray. God will get me through this!* I kept thinking.

I said very calmly, "Mother, Daddy is going to the doctor this morning, and I'm pretty sure we will get to the bottom of the problem. Is there anything I need to know or should know before we go? I'm relatively certain the doctor will recommend no driving for Daddy. Are you prepared to be the driver? This means no driver's license for him, and that means no car insurance on Daddy, so he absolutely cannot drive a car or his truck."

I decided to take this even further. "Mother, have you made out a trust? If you have, whom have you appointed as trustee of the trust and will? Who have you made the medical appointee?"

Her answer was "*You.*"

Let me take a minute here and just ask, Do you remember reading the book *The Scarlet Letter?* Remember how Hester's clothes were marked with a big *A*? I felt like the Big *U* had just been painted on my forehead. I felt like all eyes would be on me, judging *good job / bad job* or good daughter / bad daughter. Oh my, what a responsibility! I could feel the panic starting to flood my soul. My inner being wanted to run, wanted to retreat to the corner and curl up in a big ball in the fetal position and shake and blubber. I told myself to take deep breaths, to breathe, breathe deeply! I was an adult dealing with young teenage minds again.

Then I realized that this was not about me. Mother and Daddy did not choose for this to happen. This is an ugly illness. It strips everything away from their very being—their memory, their dignity. I was so sad for them, but I knew I could not break emotionally. I had work to do, things to organize, tasks to get done. I knew in my heart there would be mountains to climb, major obstacles to overcome, and that this was not going to go down easily. Again, I thought, *Be still and know I'm God! He has my back. I will get through this. I will make it. God will see me through.*

CHAPTER 5

The Old Silver Bullet Comes Home

As I look back on all the things that happened and all the decisions that we made—some good and some bad—this was definitely not one that was well thought out. The doctor reconfirmed that Daddy had Alzheimer's disease and that he was in the later stages. He agreed that Daddy did not need to operate heavy equipment or drive any type of vehicle. With that said, it would have been a perfect time for neither Daddy nor Mother to drive the car. It was in Illinois. It did not need to come home! *Perfect*! Wow! How God answered prayers!

Here is how that went wrong: (1) a situation is not thought through and (2) you don't let God be in control. I felt that the drive-off was monumental, but it was still eighteen months before we got the job done properly, getting caregivers in place. Instead, I brought the car home! I had it shipped from Illinois to Indiana!

> **"There is no second-guessing yourself in hindsight."**

Once I got it home and drove it to see how it was running, I thought, *Oh my gosh!* I was mortified that my parents were driving around in that junkyard-ready car. It had no shocks; it was awful. It had two hundred thousand miles on it. It was a death trap on wheels waiting to happen! Much later, I thought, *I had it out of state!* That was perfect. I could have said, "No, Dad, you cannot drive anymore. And, Mom, you don't need to be driving either."

But no. It was eighteen months later when we finally did take the keys from Mom. We should have had the caregivers come in at that point. They drove and took my parents everywhere. Instead, we brought the car home. Furthermore, I told my parents they needed to buy a new car, that this one was in bad shape. There was no need to put money into that old thing. Where was my brain?

Mother went out and bought a new one the next day, before I could get back up there to help them even select one. With that thoughtless decision, we were off and running for eighteen months without caregivers. It could possibly have all happened a lot easier. How will I ever know for sure? I feel there was a window of opportunity that I closed without thinking the situation through completely. However, it could have caused even more animosity with my mother than what we had. There is no way of ever knowing.

Truly, in these situations, lots of things can happen. There is no second-guessing yourself in hindsight. My advice, though, is that the best thing to do is have more communication with family, friends and professionals. The more help you can find in your decision-making, the better you will be, and it will be less stressful for everyone involved. It truly takes a village to help you take care of a person or persons with Alzheimer's disease. This was not the time to become weak. Inner strength would have to be found, and *now*!

CHAPTER 6

Red Flags

Mother was always a very neat housekeeper. The carpets were kept clean, and shoes were never to be worn on the carpet. Mother was a "take your shoes off at the door" type housekeeper. When I went to my parents' home to visit, I began to spot little things happening that were not normal. Carpet cleaner spray bottles were sitting around, and there were tar-like spots on the carpets throughout the house. Tables, chairs, pictures and keepsakes were very dusty. When I opened the refrigerator, there were numerous outdated items on the shelves, including science project leftovers with mold growing on them. It was all starting to concern me.

You must understand the people we were dealing with. They have been labeled "the Greatest Generation." They lived through the Great Depression and World War II. They raised a family during difficult times, with the heartbreaking moments of their own parents' passing.

As their child, they were not going to understand or appreciate how I could suddenly be critical of how they conducted their lives. However, we were in a crisis situation here, detrimental to their health and safety, and someone had to hit it head on.

I looked around and saw no one else. I wish there had been. No one wants to be the one to tell their parents that it's time to bring in help or it's time to investigate assisted living. This was the conversation that I had hoped would never happen. The smell in the house told the story. Someone could no longer control their bladder. I didn't dare follow the soiled carpet path to my daddy's room. One could only imagine.

At that point, I felt that I was already out of control, living in a nightmare. I was reeling from the horrified emotions, thoughts and the visual pictures. I did not want or ever think that this was how life would go for them. I had envisioned many situations I might be in with my parents as they grew old, but for some reason, Alzheimer's disease never occurred to me as a possibility.

"They have been labeled "the Greatest Generation."

I'm the youngest of three children. I have an older sister and an older brother. Mother and Daddy appointed me as the trustee of the estate and medical appointee. When I found out I was the trustee, I called both siblings, and the conversation was as follows:

"I may have the control, but I believe we are in this situation together. This is not going to be easy. We will discuss things, sometimes vote on decisions, and the majority will rule. I will listen to everything you have to say, but sometimes all three of us may have entirely different opinions. If that is the case, I will make a decision. Sometimes we may have to agree to disagree. The money in the estate is Mother and Daddy's. It will go for their care and anything that is needed for them. It is their money and their money only, not ours to fight over. I feel we will do what we have to do."

They both were quite easy to talk to, and I could feel they respected what I had to say. Deep down, I think they were both very relieved. My brother lives out of state, and my sister has health concerns of her own. I could not have two better people to be my brother and sister. Both were always there for support and were so agreeable. They never made my job hard. We had great communication.

My brother, Jim, lives a thousand miles from Mother and Daddy, but if I asked him for help or if he could please come home, he was there in a couple of days. He is married to an awesome woman, and I know that a couple of times it had to be hard on their household for him to be gone for a week to ten days. When one parent is away, it makes it difficult for the other parent left to do it all alone, with boys still in high school and with school activities going on. My sister-in-law also works outside the home, which had to make the situation even more hectic at times. When my brother was away, his family never complained. I thank my brother for his insight, thoughts and help. I'm not sure I could have made it through without him.

My sister, Janet, is a lovely woman who would always lend an ear and give her thoughts. Yet she was always respectful of her younger sister. I could not ask for a better family. Mother and Daddy always came first in anything we did, anything we decided. They would have been enormously proud of the three of us.

CHAPTER 7

Time to Bring in the Forces

Our family is not large by any means, with only three siblings. When I was growing up, I always wished I had siblings closer to my age. My sister is almost ten years older than me, and my brother is six years older than me. As the youngest one, I never felt close to them. We were going through different stages of our lives at different times. When I was twelve years old, my sister was newly married, and I was just starting my teens. That is a big difference. My brother was in college, and we had nothing in common.

I always felt like an only child. Mother and Daddy were exceptionally good parents. We were so close and did lots of things together. Daddy loved basketball and had played in high school. I was a cheerleader all through school. Mother and Daddy always went to every game. They were always with me.

> **"I knew this conversation was going in a whole different direction."**

I missed closeness with my siblings and did not have much communication with them over the years. There were no problems between us, just the age differences. We were all at different points in our lives. My brother had moved with his wife and family to San Antonio, Texas. They were busy raising three boys. I married and moved here and there, raising my daughter and son. Just keeping up with daily routines does not leave a lot of time to share. Geographic distances do not help with closeness either, especially in the days before cell phones and the Internet.

All of us seemed to have a decent relationship with Mother and Daddy. Mother would always tell if she had heard from one of us to the other when we would call her. That way we kept up with news of each other's lives.

Now it was time to call my brother. I always enjoyed talking with my brother. He is an intelligent man, very charming and easy to talk to. He always has some funny stories to tell, and I love to hear him laugh. His laughter is infectious, and I always looked forward to our conversations. However, I knew this conversation was going in a whole different direction.

I was calling to let him know we had problems. I telephoned him, and I let him know I was seeing some changes in Mother and Daddy, just little things now, nothing major. He, of course, was thankful I called and gave him this heads-up, and he wanted to stay on top of the situation. We promised to stay in touch, and we would work together to take care of Mother and Daddy.

CHAPTER 8

The Ugly Comes Out

I'm not proud of the ugly moments in this journey, but they are part of it. Today I'm still ashamed of my reaction to a couple of situations I was in with my parents. I know in my heart now that I did not have all the information. I did not recognize that Mother was having trouble as well. I was concentrating on Daddy. I completely missed how dementia was taking Mother down too. She seemed in control, but I failed to see how bad off she really was. Still, my reaction was not good, and no one should ever lose control the way I did.

> **"This insidious disease was sucking the life out of them, and me."**

Daddy had driven off several months before. At that time, Mother was still taking care of Daddy the best she could. I had hinted at someone coming in and helping, of hiring a caregiver so Mother didn't have to do it all by herself. That suggestion fell on deaf ears. Mother would have nothing to do with that idea. It was a while after the drive off that I started noticing more and more things that were not right at Mother and Daddy's home. They were wearing the same clothes over and over. They both had a closetful, but they were wearing the same slacks and shirts every time I saw them. They never smelled dirty nor were the clothes dirty, but never different, always the same ones. There was an odor at times, but I wasn't sure. Then other times, the smell of urine was overwhelming. There were tar-like spots on the carpet, and you could find a path down the hall to the door of Dad's room.

I was the baby of the family. Yes, I was a grown woman, having raised a family of my own. However, I was raised to respect people's belongings and to honor someone's privacy. In my mind, this especially applies to your parents' home. Parents were to be revered and respected, placed up above everyone. This is how my parents were toward their own parents. You didn't dare question. Or was it really that I was scared to death as to what I would find on the other side of that door? There has been a lengthy pause in my writing because this is one part of the book I'm not particularly proud of. It has been extremely difficult to put down on paper. The anger I felt inside was at times out of control, not that I showed it or expressed it outwardly. Inside, I was in emotional turmoil, not knowing or understanding the *why*. Not having any answers, the heartbreak of watching two wonderful people disintegrate before my eyes was horrifying. This insidious disease was sucking the life out of them, and me. I decided my brother needed to come home to help me address Mother and Daddy about the need for help to come in. When he did, we met with my sister first. Talking among ourselves, we each shared moments where we had seen changes in both our parents. We agreed that things were getting extremely hard for Mother to take care of by herself. We decided it was time for all of us to sit down together and have this conversation with Mother and Daddy.

We began by telling our parents we loved them and cared and wanted to help. We always teased my brother through the years that being the only boy, he was Mom's favorite, so he should be the spokesman. He started out not by attacking but mentioning some things that seemed to be getting out of control. He pointed out the spots on the floor and both of them wearing the same clothes over and over again. He remarked on Mother's hair being long, oily and stringy. (This was a major difference in itself, because Mother had her hair done once a week and was always dressed very well.) Mother and Daddy always said it didn't matter what you had as long as you kept it clean and always put forth your best. Their appearances were totally different than they had ever been. He also talked about outdated items in the fridge, about Daddy driving off, various dents in the car, etc.

Let's just say it did not go well. Mother let us know in no uncertain terms that she was in control and that she did not ask for our help. She stated vehemently that we should just mind our own business! The hateful claws came out toward us all, but it did seem like they were aimed toward her beloved son more than anyone. *Wow*! She was mad! This was a side of our mother that no one had ever seen!

All of us looked at Dad, and all he had to say was "Whatever your mother wants."

With that said, I wanted to calm this down. It was obvious to us we had a major problem, but the situation needed to cool down for the moment. I stated, "Let's do this for now: Let's give it six weeks."

I prayed silently, *God, get us through this and let's think about this some more!*

Then I suggested that after six weeks, we would look at the situation again and go from there. If there were any more problems, *then* help would come in.

"Mother and Daddy," I said, "you have put me in charge. You trusted that I would make the right decisions for your well-being. I am afraid that time has come, and we will make changes as we need to."

I couldn't believe some of the things that came out of my mouth, as I was calm, businesslike and not at all emotional! It was not anything at all like how I was feeling.

I did have the forethought (even though we had hit a brick wall for the moment) to go ahead and contact the caregiver who I was most interested in. I put her in a sort of stand-by mode. Later, I was so glad that I had. It was in mid-September, a few weeks after that initial talk, that I felt the need to check out my dad's bedroom. Lord, have mercy! This inspection would have told us the whole story if one of us would have checked this out years before that September day. The reason I say years is because there is no way that room could have gotten in that condition in just a few months.

What I found was terrifying and sickening. Daddy's room was in shambles—the bed, the floor. I stood in disbelief. The strong smell of urine permeated the room. The carpet had huge spots of feces everywhere. When I uncovered the bed, there was a rotted-out hole in the mattress the size of a gallon bucket. I looked at my mother in horror. At that moment, I felt as if I was in a medieval mental ward looking at someone sleeping in their own urine and feces.

All I could say, as I was holding back my tears, was "Mother! *Why*?"

Mother said to me, "It is awful, isn't it?"

I said, "Yes, it certainly is."

I knew then that Mother was sick. She was very, very sick!

I stood there with my phone in my hand and started making calls. Carpet cleaners came the next day. I had the bed and mattress hauled out. I ordered a new bed, sheets, blankets, new underwear, disposable underwear and pajamas for Daddy. Within twenty-four hours, things were cleaned up. I stayed the week, going home at night after making sure Dad was wearing disposable underwear. I put him to bed with pillows around him and a blow-up mattress on the floor, so if he fell out, he would land on it and not hurt himself.

During the day, I cleaned out the cabinets, pitching outdated cereal and canned goods. I remember that while I was doing this, Mother got mad because I was throwing everything out. How wasteful!

I told her, "There is a whole garbage bag full of outdated cereal. I'll put it over in the corner for you, but Dad and I will be eating the good stuff!"

She then decided it was okay to throw it out.

The dust around the baseboards was thick. I found sheets in the dryer that smelled like urine. I knew we needed caregivers immediately, but how could I do it with Mother's staunch objections? This had been on my mind since our conversation with them. I knew we had to get this done. I prayed for God to open a door somehow. I could only do so much. My husband and I owned a business, and I also had a full-time job working for the county. I wasn't Wonder Woman after all.

My husband and I owned a sporting goods business, and bow season for deer is in October. We loved to hunt on Mother and Daddy's farm. We had plans to go up and hunt one day, and I had told Mother we would be there at 9:00 a.m. We had several things going on that morning, and we were not able to make it by then, so I called Mother and told her we were going to be late.

She just said okay.

We finally made it there at about 10:45 a.m., and when we arrived, Daddy was lying on the family room floor. He seemed disoriented.

I asked Mother, "How long has he been on the floor like this?"

Her answer was "I don't know."

This was when the dam broke. I broke!

In a demanding tone, I said, "You live in this house and you can't tell me how long Daddy has been lying here on this floor? I don't believe that, Mother! Now answer my question. How long has he been on the floor?"

She said, "Oh, all right, he's been there all night."

I screamed, "All *night*? Are you trying to *kill him, Mother*? He is a diabetic. Has he had his meds, water or food? What the hell, *Mother*? I called you this morning and you said nothing about a problem. You have my phone number. You could have called us last night, and you know we would have been here immediately. As of now, Mother, you will no longer take care of him! I will have caregivers here today, as fast as I can get them here. You are done!"

I was in shock. I was pissed. I was heartbroken for both Daddy and Mother. So many thoughts and pictures flooded my mind. I could visualize it as sparks flying, hitting the brain. I wanted to short-circuit. Alzheimer's, memory loss, dementia, the changes in them, the lost look in their eyes, the repeated stories, the poop on the carpet, dents in the car, the not talking. I realized I wasn't only dealing with one sick parent. I was dealing with two. Several years before, I was friends with a lady at work who had to hire caregivers to take care of her parents. On break time, I would overhear Debbie talking to the caregivers on the phone. There were many conversations about different subjects like bathing, meals and taking rides. I heard Debbie call one of the caregivers by the name Elizabeth. This stuck in my mind. From what I could gather, this Elizabeth was awesome. I wanted to hire Elizabeth.

I got her number, and we had a genuinely nice phone conversation. I had called her back in September with hopes that our first conversation with Mother and Daddy would go well and that help would start then. I had warned her that she might not be starting to work with us until later. I also told her that I understood if another offer came along that she might have to take it, but I really wanted her. I was trying my hardest to get the job done. She was very understanding. She said that it had been her experience that when the family gets to this point, it may take a few weeks, but it will happen.

Elizabeth is one in a million. She had been with the last couple for three years. She has twenty years of caregiving experience. She has been through it all. The woman is remarkable. In many of our conversations, she helped me to grow in attitude. She shared many thoughts, but most of all, she wanted me to let go of the caregiving part and be the daughter. She could see that was hard for me to do.

In the beginning, I thought I was some kind of Wonder Woman. I had a "I can do it all" attitude. After all, these were my parents. I knew what I wanted for them. I knew the care I wanted for them. I just needed help. I had a mission to make them *well*. Elizabeth had a great sense of humor, and that is the only thing that kept her from killing me.

CHAPTER 9

The Real Wonder Woman

From the point of Elizabeth taking control and me answering to her, things only continued to get better. She began by hiring only the best. We went through a few unacceptable hires at first, but she weeded out the ones that did not perform the duties that were expected of them. Elizabeth expected a journal to be kept on every shift. It was pretty simple to write in a notebook the duties that were performed daily or nightly. If it was not recorded in the book, then it didn't happen.

For example, medications taken. She had a simple form for meds, which ones and what time they were given. Dinner was at what time, what did the meal consist of, how much was consumed. Shower was given or not, and if not, why was it not given. Also, the condition of the skin was to be reported. Did the skin have a rash, redness or marks of any kind? Exercise daily, a walk around the property. Even when the weather was inclement, Elizabeth would make sure they had walks inside as well. She made sure everyone knew what was expected in caring for Mr. and Mrs. Williams.

Your name was in that book, and you signed off after your shift. It was like a Bible. She wanted every detail. It made everyone accountable. When you have caregivers, you need everyone doing their jobs. Staff could explain why something didn't get done, but when you don't have accountability, then sometimes a small problem becomes a larger problem fast.

Time is important in dealing with elderly people. It is too fragile; they are too fragile. A small cut or scratch or sore can become infected before you know it. However, when someone reported that Mr. Williams had a small scratch on his arm, it could be taken care of immediately. If a caregiver did not know a procedure to follow, then calling Elizabeth was advised. Her goal was that everyone communicated with each other and with the journal. This was a most professional approach.

> **"When you have caregivers, you need everyone doing their jobs."**

Elizabeth came in with a mission, and that was to make the end of life the absolute best it could possibly be for my parents. She would not settle for less. From the condition of the house to Daddy's skin condition to his feet, shaving, their meds, food, exercise and their daily rides. Every day she had a project, and that project came before anything else.

We studied how things were getting done and how we could improve the conditions of the situation. Daddy's bed was one issue. Was he sleeping, was it wet or dry, could he fall out, was it kept clean and were the sheets changed regularly? I'm one for making a job easier. Bed rails were suggested, but Elizabeth pointed out that an AD patient could get a leg or arm caught in those, and it could cause a terrible injury. She was in a panic when I suggested moving the bed against the wall so there would be one side he couldn't fall out of. A body pillow was placed against the wall. That was softer to hit than the wall. She agreed with that, and an air mattress was placed on the floor so that side was softer to hit than the floor.

Her panic was because it would be more difficult to clean and change the sheets. I asked if she had ever heard of furniture sliders. A puzzled look on her face told me she had never heard of them. I told her I would get some and she would be able to slide that bed with one finger. She looked at me like I had lost my mind. I ran up to the local chain store and could not get back to the house fast enough to show her how easy it would be. She was totally amazed. It was so easy to slide!

Elizabeth and I, and sometimes my brother, would have brainstorming sessions on how situations could be made easier. I was determined to keep Mother and Daddy in their home as long as possible, and that we did. As they became more and more unbalanced, belts were used to help them to the bathroom and shower.

Soon we discovered that the bathroom would have to be enlarged to accommodate two people, both the caregiver and Daddy or Mother. That was no problem. The handyman was soon called, and the bathroom was enlarged. Elizabeth soon found out that anything for our parents' comfort would be discussed, figured out, planned and finished without hesitation.

We wanted them to remain in their home as promised. The discussion with my mother was that I would keep them on the farm as long as they knew where they were. The days and weeks changed the house a lot. It became a hustle-bustle type place. The living room was Daddy's place, where he could watch Westerns on TV or listen to Hank Williams on the stereo or where he and Elizabeth could talk. Oh, how they talked! She would engage my father in many conversations about farming, horses, buggies, family, how he grew up, basketball, World War II stories and on and on.

Elizabeth also tried every day to get them outside for a walk. My daddy loved the outdoors, so they often took walks down the lane or back to the pond. Sometimes they walked out to the carriage house. I think that was one of Daddy's favorite places to go. She would help him walk out there, and they would look around. Sometimes it was as if he had never seen it all before, and he would be in awe. Sometimes he remembered an item, and then he would look for it, almost like a game. Then sometimes he didn't remember that these things belonged to him.

Other days, he enjoyed showing the carriages to Elizabeth, as she said that the carriages were beautiful, and she loved looking at them as well. She remembered one day though that Daddy wanted her to sit in one (I always called it the Cinderella carriage), and Dad shut the door. That happened to be the one you couldn't open from the inside.

"*Wow*! That was a little frightening for a few minutes," Elizabeth told me later. "But thank goodness your dad remembered how to open the door!"

Daddy told her, "You didn't need to worry. I wouldn't let anything happen to you."

Daddy was old-school. Elizabeth and I witnessed that one day taking him to the doctor's office. The man could barely walk, but he held the door open for Elizabeth, myself and another lady who was walking in. (He may have forgotten a lot, but he remembered gentlemanly manners!)

The lady thanked Daddy and commented, "You just don't see much of that anymore, men being gentlemen."

Daddy just smiled.

Elizabeth also made videos for me. On my father's passing, she gave me one she had made of him waving at me and telling me, "Hi!" I love it. It means the world to me. Jenny was one of the night shift caregivers. She had a closeness with both Mother and Daddy, and she also made some touching videos. Sometimes in the night, if one of them was having trouble getting to sleep or having a restless night, she would sit with them. Sometimes, she sat, just talking about the day or passing days or maybe reading to them poetry or short stories. She did anything to relax them and help them to fall asleep.

Ms. Sherry was Mother's caregiver, and she took particularly good care of Mother. Mother would go outside sometimes, but not often. Before the caregivers took over, Mother had become so quiet in her decline, and she had a strict routine that she kept too. She was so strict about the routine that the house had become a tomb. She insisted that the TV be on only in the evening. No radio, no talking, hardly anything to eat. Meds were only taken when she remembered, which wasn't often.

Elizabeth came in and flipped things around and upside down. The *new* routine included cooking using the crock pot, washing clothes, showers daily with moisturizer used after the showers, disposable underwear was used when needed, comfortable clothes were to be worn.

The closet doors were opened, and Elizabeth was told to use every article of clothing. If items become soiled or stained, Elizabeth was to throw them away. Mother had kept wearing the same three outfits over and over. I explained to her that there was no need for that because everything in that closet could not be worn or worn out in twenty years of time! So use it all!

Elizabeth made sure that Ms. Sherry and some of the other caregivers understood the clothing was to be used. Ms. Sherry and Elizabeth made sure Mother looked good again, wearing pretty slacks and tops, with her hair combed and fixed. It was nice seeing Mother looking cared for.

Lift chairs were purchased for both of them. We bought new blankets that were warm and fuzzy. There were snacks and sweets, fruit and water, water, water. We gave them water in special glasses with packets of lemonade or tea flavors—anything to get the water down.

There was nothing that my parents wanted for. The caregivers took them on a ride every day and sometimes two rides. Mother and Daddy both loved to ride, and we suspect the rides would end with some kind of ice cream treat. (But those were secret treats, making them all the more special!)

Elizabeth called hospice, and we worked closely with them. We thought we had a good hospice organization locally, but it wasn't until Mother and Daddy were admitted into the nursing home that I truly became aware of how awesome hospice was. Elizabeth made the three-year period as comfortable as possible for them. None of it was easy for anyone. She truly put her heart and soul into their care. The Williams family took care of Elizabeth too, and she is thought of as part of our family today. She is Wonder Woman. She is in a class of her own.

CHAPTER 10

The Day of Reckoning

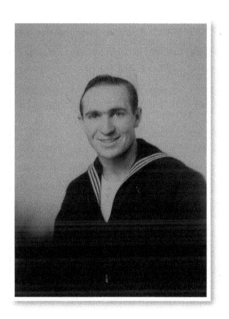

Hiring caregivers is sometimes a surrender. It means admitting that you can no longer be beneficial to the health and well-being of the other party. I felt like I was betraying my daddy and mother. Mother and I had a conversation about the state of affairs after the family meeting. I had thought a lot about the caregiving and how badly they both needed it. But when you are dealing with people who are called "The Greatest Generation," it is exceedingly difficult to get the smallest of jobs done when it pertains to their care.

I remember Tom Brokow, news commentator and writer, who wrote in his book that these were young people, like all of us at a young age, who have dreams and hopes but are fighting a world war. It didn't matter what part of the earth you were on; it was in turmoil. These were the people that had gone through rough times in the Great Depression, who didn't have food or heat. Sometimes their parents didn't have jobs; they were extremely poor.

My parents were in all those conditions growing up. When my daddy was eighteen and graduated from high school, he, like a lot of young men in that era, joined the service. He told many stories of being in the Navy. What was very strange to me was that Dad always made it sound like "Yeah, we fought some battles." *Some* battles! He fought in the Pacific War Battle of Okinawa. He was a gunner on the ship and said he shot down a few suicide bomber planes that flew near. As a matter of fact, the Japanese suicide planes were so close at times, he could see the pilot's eyes.

I was always amazed. I asked Daddy one time, "Daddy, didn't you feel scared, and didn't you just want it all to stop? The noise, the bombs, day and night, didn't you feel like you couldn't do it anymore? Didn't you just want it to stop and for it all to go away? Weren't you homesick? Didn't you just want to be on the farm again?"

Dad kind of shrugged his shoulders and said, "Sure, you always thought about home, the younger kids, Mom and Daddy. You even thought back to the hunting dogs, just everything goes through your mind."

He said he had a job to do, and a lot of people were depending on him. He had three meals a day and a bed to sleep in. He was the second of nine children, and things at home were tight.

He said, "Why, shooting those planes was nothing. Those were big guns."

He said he thought there was no missing with those big guns, that he had a system and it worked.

It must have been a good system, because he came home and had a wonderful, blessed life. Very independent people, "The Greatest Generation." They made their way in life; they had the feeling that they had survived. Through all the ugly, danger and hardship in life, they had taken care of living, and they would continue to do so.

Now their youngest daughter was taking control of their life, and I was resented for it. When I stepped in, I was taking Mother's place. Mother still had enough recognition of the situation that she was bitter, annoyed and resentful. One had to remember that the marriage of my parents was a lengthy one—sixty-eight years. Many commitments and promises were made to each other over that span of time. One promise was until death do us part. I know they promised to never put one another in a nursing home.

When Mother and I had our heart-to-heart talk after the family conversation, and after Daddy was left on the floor all night, I had been up all night figuring out how this was to be approached. I have to say my brain was taxed. My emotions were drained. Decisions had to be made. Winter was coming, and they could not be up there on the hill back that long lane another winter without help.

I went in that morning to Mother and Daddy's, poised and in control. I had a plan, and now the plan would be put in motion. It was the day of reckoning, as my father would have said. Too many people were depending on me.

I said to Mother, "Do you remember when you and Daddy bought this property, all of the briars and weeds and thorn trees that were cleared to build this beautiful home and farm you have? Mom, half of this farm is Daddy's, and half of all accounts are Daddy's. Whatever it takes to help Dad and you get through this, then that is what we will spend Daddy's share of the money on—help for him. What I will do today is get an account of all assets, and if we need to sell half of the farm acreages to maintain him here, then this is what shall be done.

"You are very tired," I continued. "And you need rest and help with Daddy. Today at twelve noon, caregivers will come in to help you and Daddy. They will cook, clean, bathe Daddy and take you on your afternoon ride. We will see how it works. With them here during the day and putting Daddy to bed and leaving at eight p.m., this should help you get some badly needed rest."

She wasn't happy, but she didn't argue with me about half the money being Dad's and him being taken care of and her being tired. I really think she thought she could be mean enough, and no one would stay working for her. She truly underestimated me and Elizabeth. I'm a chip off the old block, and Elizabeth has been doing this for many, many years. Her years of experience helped Elizabeth through.

Poor Elizabeth! Not only did she have to take care of Dad and build a trust with him, she had to get Mother in a frame of mind of accepting and building a trust with her as well. Good Lord, she was also going to have to take Wonder Woman (*me!*) down a notch or two. Or take Wonder Woman behind the buggy shed and kick her butt. That's who I thought I was—Wonder Woman! I was Johnny-on-the-spot with supplies, food or whatever was needed. Elizabeth wanted for nothing when it came to material things to make the job easier.

Elizabeth knew I had a problem with accepting how this illness was going. She could see it in me when she told me on the phone, "Your dad is doing great! We had such a good talk or walk!"

Then I would come, and he would be out of it, with a lost look in his eyes. I would be extremely disappointed. I wanted the same. I wanted his talking, I wanted the walking, I wanted the laughing, I wanted my dad back!

When I acted like that, I made Elizabeth feel unappreciated, and she thought I was unsatisfied with all the work she was doing. This was very upsetting to her because there were so many things that had been out of order, like their meds, for one. Neither one of them had been taking their meds correctly. She said it was a wonder either one was alive.

Mother would get up in the morning and turn the skillet on and forget it. Toenails were horrible and untrimmed. Doctor appointments were haphazardly kept, or not at all. Those are just a few of the things that had to be straightened out. The list of things went on and on.

Elizabeth would tell me how good Dad was, then she would be off for a few days, and he did not respond to the other caregivers as he did her. I would panic. I would call her and tell her that he was doing badly. She would go check on him, and of course he was better when she was there.

Elizabeth knew that Wonder Woman needed a reality check. She was waiting for the right time. She knew I would be upset and that it would be devastating for me. It had been a couple of months, and we had gone through a few caregivers. One evening, my brother called and we were talking, and he started telling me that I should be a manager, not a caregiver.

I had shared with him about being at Mom and Dad's when a caregiver had quit, and I went for the evening. I put Dad in bed and mentioned changing Dad's disposable underwear.

My brother went ballistic. He said, "No one ever expected you to do those jobs, sis. Of course, this is heartbreaking. But Janet and I never expected you to be the one to perform those kinds of duties.

"You need to be the manager," he went on. "Overseeing but not actually *performing* the caregiving! I appreciate everything you are doing, Teresa, but Dad would not want you or Janet to do that. And to be honest, I could *not* do it. We may have to put Dad in a nursing home if we can't keep the help."

I have to say that when I got off the phone with him, I was frustrated and upset too. I thought, *I'm here. What the hell or who in the hell is going to do those jobs?*

Shortly after that, Elizabeth and I were having a conversation, and she was sharing with me how Dad was doing and how good he was responding. I will never forget that day and the phrase she used when all the lights came on upstairs for me.

"He is doing good for the situation we are in!" she stated.

I took a deep breath and finally realized that I would never make him well. I could not work miracles. Nor would there be any phenomenal breakthrough performed by Elizabeth, or any doctor or nurse or any other caregivers. AD had him, and it would take him down. Keep him comfortable, keep him clean and safe, well fed, help him save some dignity, keep him happy and smiling.

In realizing the situation that we were in, I also realized that I was not the one who needed to be the manager. Let's face it, I was good at managing people. My background was business owner. I had owned several different small businesses. However, I knew nothing about the business of caregiving. I didn't even know the questions to ask when hiring one, and that was obvious because of the turnover we had experienced for a few weeks.

It came to me that I had a woman, Elizabeth, with twenty years of experience who knew what to look for. I gave her a raise and made her the manager of that household. I told her to hire the very best, and I told her the budget we had. She was so happy that I stepped out of her way, and she started taking control immediately and making adjustments.

I would say that for home health care, we had one of the best teams in the state. I was impressed with her control and the decisions she was making for Daddy and Mother's care and health. I felt that at some point, she needed to start her own business. She is that awesome. This is exactly where she thought I needed to be with her as well—that she was the only one answering to me, and I was finally being the daughter. She thought that was the only role I needed to have. She thought I sucked at being Wonder Woman! And I did.

CHAPTER 11

Silver Hair, Golden Heart

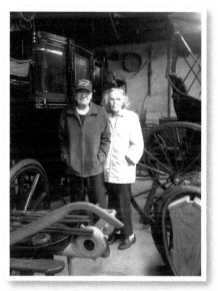

One of the most beautiful women I have ever known is an older lady, thinly built, silver hair, clothing very formfitting, precise. It is an unusual friendship. I met her at the bank. Through the years, she handled our business accounts. I always enjoyed talking to her. Bretta is also a member of the same church we attended, where she plays the piano every Sunday morning. Bretta is a mild-mannered woman, very much in control of her thinking and her speaking. She is very classy in the way she handles herself.

When my parents became sick, I started finding accounts. I sought Bretta out for help. My parents had used that bank since the beginning of their time together, more than sixty years. Bretta was vice president and was immensely helpful. I was totally unaware of the accounts my parents had and the amounts. She was instrumental in setting up a checking account with my name added. In her years at the bank, she had run into many unusual family situations, and nothing surprised her—from families not getting along to accounts that the family knew nothing about. The list of financial issues was endless.

I approached her about my parents being ill and how I had been appointed the trustee of their estate. I have to say, I probably had a very bewildered look on my face. She knew instantly how to guide me forward. She had information she shared to ensure that every-thing was done legally. She was wonderful and wonderful to talk to.

As my parents' illnesses progressed, I looked at their estate in awe. I couldn't believe the size of the estate they had and that they had done nothing to prepare for this time in their lives. They had been collectors of antiques, carriages and many, many other items. I realized that they enjoyed them. It wasn't about the money. One would say it was about the find, the quest. It was fun for them to go each day for a different drive and locate items. They collected those antiques and put them in their buildings for show, for them and others to see and enjoy.

There were stories behind the carriages or the baby bed and where they found each item. They remembered the sale or auction they had attended to find this or that. These were fun times for them, I'm sure. I never heard how much it all cost. It was about how you used it or how it was used back in the day that mattered. That meant *their* day of growing up or their parents' days of growing up. I always found each story fascinating. As I looked upon what we had, I was scared. I was unsure of how we would sell this amazing collection and how we would keep it safe until that time came. It was mind-bog-gling. It was a huge undertaking.

I went into the bank one day on personal business, and of course Miss Bretta was at her desk. I sat down, and we talked about my personal banking. And then she asked if everything was okay. I asked her if she knew anything about estate business.

She said, "Yes, some. I have worked with people over the years on their estates."

"I need help!" I exclaimed quite simply.

Bretta said, "Okay, honey, what can I do?"

With that opening, I poured it out to her. I said, "Daddy has a buggy shed full of antiques, and the house is full, and I have no idea what I'm going to do! Would you go with me sometime just to take a look and tell me what you think?"

She agreed, and we set a date for her to go with me to survey the situation.

Let's step back to the beginning of that conversation. I called it a buggy shed. I'm sure this created a picture in her mind—or anyone else's—that my parents lived on a farm down some gravel road out in the boonies somewhere. She had no idea what she was walking into. Did she envision a few antiques out in a dilapidated old building out in a hog lot somewhere? I sounded like a country girl raised by an old country boy calling our outbuildings sheds. That paints a whole different picture for someone other than the reality of the situation. We drove to the south edge of what looked like a medium-sized city. There were paved roads off a major state highway.

Bretta had told me that in her spare time, she worked for the best auctioneer in the state. I was elated to hear this because this is how it works: if Bretta tells you something, you can take it to the bank. (No pun intended. Okay, yes, it was intended!) She is solid, she is truthful, her word is good.

I felt like I was making progress. I had the treasurer of an auction company with me at this point, and I felt enthralled with every word that was coming out of her mouth. As we were riding along, she said that having an auction sale is sometimes hard because of the location. Sometimes the roads are gravel, or the place is off the beaten path and hard to find. She said that so far, all this looked great—highway most of the way and a paved road to the house.

Then we arrived. We drove up an exceptionally long lane, with a black-topped drive part of the way. We stopped in front of a red brick building and a beautiful red brick home. Out beyond the house stood a huge red and white metal building with hills and fields surrounding us. It was not your rundown muddy horse or pig lot that she might have conjured in her mind because of this country girl's use of the English language!

Daddy's buggy shed indeed! As I watched her face, I asked her if we could go in while we were there, and I would introduce her to my parents. I warned her that they would not talk much, and they probably wouldn't remember that we'd even been there. I explained that I always made myself known, and I always checked in with my caregivers in case anyone needed anything.

As we went in, everyone was bustling around as the morning routine was in progress. Elizabeth was rubbing my father's feet with lotion as he had just been bathed, and they were in deep conversation about farming. Mother was eating a midmorning snack. She had already been bathed, dressed and had her hair fixed. She looked so nice, and all seemed calm.

Later, they would be going for their afternoon ride, which they both enjoyed. Most of the time, it consisted of some kind of ice cream. (Not one time would the caregivers admit to stopping and getting ice cream, and I loved the caregivers for it. They cared for them so much that they were treating them special, and that warmed my heart!) I knew they were doing this, and I always made sure the cash was there for these special things.

I introduced Miss Bretta to everyone and told my folks I was showing Miss Bretta the carriage house and the collections. With that done, off we went.

As we walked out of the house, Bretta was concentrating on the large metal barn. We walked toward my van, which was parked in front of this rather large red brick building, pillars in front, with a cement porch. We reached the door of the building, and I turned to her and said, "I hope you can help. I really need to know what I need to do."

When I opened the door, the look on her face was priceless. She looked above in the rafters and then at all the carriages—seventeen of them housed in this building. She swayed from side to side and, in a breathless voice, just kept saying, "*My, oh, my!*" Then she turned and walked down a small side aisle and was quiet. Then again, she would say, "*Oh, my! My, my, my! Oh my! Oh, honey!*" She said, "Teresa, this collection is one that there are no words for."

As I looked around, I saw everything from apple cider presses, baskets of books, stone crocks, lanterns, old signage. The building was packed with antiques. Again, Bretta sighed. Mother and Daddy were not pack rats. Every antique that they had bought had been wiped down and polished. Nothing had been altered. Usually cleaning was the extent of their efforts. Then each item found a home somewhere in the buggy shed, either in the rafters, hanging on the walls or placed on shelves. The carriages were side by side, ready for driving. Harnesses for the horses were with each carriage. Every carriage and harness was polished and ready for the next parade.

Bretta admitted to me later that it was nothing like she had imagined. She thought we were going out to the big red metal building. She said, "Teresa, this is like a museum. Everything in here is of museum quality. By no means am I saying that the company I am with is the only one that can do this sale." She continued, "I do feel that Mr. Boston always does a great job. He advertises his sales well, and he gets the most he can out of everything auctioned. The first thing we need to do is decide if an auction is how you want to go."

I had told her earlier that security was my main concern. Once Daddy and Mother were off the property and the house was empty, it would only be a matter of time before it would be broken into and destroyed. I could not let that happen. She suggested that if I wanted Mr. Boston to do this, he would need to come and see it.

"Then let's make an appointment with him!" I replied.

Within a few days Mr. Boston called me, and I took him up to the building to show him the collection. Even though Bretta had spoken with him about the collections, his reaction was still surprised when I opened the door. There was more than he had anticipated, and the museum quality of the items was mind-boggling. Not too many times in his years of auctions had he seen antiques of such fine quality. He felt he could do a great job for us.

Over several months of talking and planning, we decided that a sale of the household items, a few antiques, barn items, tractors and lawn mowers would be held first. That sale in itself was huge. He told me that when the time came to move my parents to the nursing home, we could then plan the auctions a few weeks after that, and we did.

Moving day came. The house was going to sit empty, which scared me. I just didn't want it vandalized, robbed or windows broken out. The location of the farm is beautiful, but it does sit back that long lane, and it is isolated back there. It was a perfect place for lots of bad things to happen. Having that worry as my forethought, I was in a hurry to get it cleaned out.

My daughter and I cleaned and moved things to the garage. Going through fifty years of life, through my parents' lives, just seemed odd, surreal. Sorting through pictures and private notes was difficult, but we got through it. I think the hardest of all was the clothing Mother and Daddy had, and they both were blessed with a lot. The smell of them and remembering how they looked when an item was worn touched my heart. The dress worn to my second marriage, the blouse worn to Mom's fortieth wedding anniversary, the suit Daddy wore to my wedding. Ties! It goes on and on and it hurts. When you discard those items, it feels like you are discarding them. You want to go back to those times and relive those moments. You realize they are never going to be there again, and the memories are all you have.

On the mantle of the fireplace was a small lantern with a handle on it, and also the irons that were warmed on a Warm Morning stove when my mother was a little girl. Mother called it an ice skater's light lantern. It was carried by someone when they ice skated in the evening. I always found that to be strange, the idea of someone skating at night when it was cold, yet the picture in my mind was beautiful. I imagined a little girl with a scarf, gloves and a petite coat on, reminding me of Currier and Ives postcards.

Mother told me that when she was a little girl, there were four children in her family. They were extremely poor during that time, and there was very little heat in the house. She told about her mother warming the irons on the Warm Morning stove, wrapping them in towels when they would get warm and putting them under the covers at the end of the bed to keep their feet warm. All four of the children slept in the same bed. I was always intrigued with such items, and the stories behind them were so fascinating to me. Those are the types of items I have kept, and someday I will pass them on to my children and grandchildren.

My son and his wife, Emely, came as well and helped for a few days. Without both of those families coming and helping me, I'm not sure I could have gotten the job done by myself. I had trouble getting past the private part of it all, the respect you have been taught through the years. This was my parents' home, and there is a reverence about that. Now all of a sudden, they were not there, and it was okay to go through their stuff.

All that was going through my mind, and at times the grief was so overwhelming that I felt like I was a china plate that could shatter into a million pieces if it was placed wrong or bumped just so. You feel very fragile. B-o-o-t-s-t-r-a-p-s! Bootstraps. You find them and you pull yourself up. You have a job to do, and you must get the job done somehow, some way, because that is what your parents expected you to do.

After the first auction, my partner for years in law enforcement agreed to take care of security on the farm. He and his wife lived in the house and took care of everything, ensuring that the items in the carriage house would remain safe. I couldn't have asked for a better solution because he and his wife are the best people ever! I walked in the house one time to get some items out of it and looked curiously around. I asked my husband if they were still living in the house because it was so clean it didn't look occupied! You can't find better people than that. Joe and his wife were a Godsend to us.

But I am getting ahead of myself. Mother and Daddy were in the nursing home, never coming back, when I decided to get the first sale out of the way. Then my father passed the week before that sale took place. I was devastated. My heart broke. This was not how this was supposed to happen. I felt that I was being so disrespectful, that just one week after he passed away, we were having a sale. I was sick. Did we look like vultures to the community? I felt like everyone was saying, "He's not even cold and she is selling everything."

I had honored my parents all my life, and this was terrifying to me. Mr. Boston knew my heart was breaking and understood the embarrassment I felt. He took total control the morning of the auction and opened with a speech about how this sale had been planned weeks before the passing of Mr. Williams. Once the fliers and the advertising went out, it would have been hard to retract and reschedule.

He further explained that this was not what the family had anticipated, and if they had, this sale would certainly not have been happening that day. He asked the crowd to please understand our heartbreak.

As my dear friend, the silver-haired lady Bretta had said, Jeff Boston is the best, and she was right. I was surrounded by lots of wonderful people that day, not that it kept my heart from breaking to see a lifetime of items, furniture and memories walk off the farm. But I was comforted by knowing that people cared and felt my pain as well.

Upon my father's passing, I remember driving home from the nursing home that evening. The funeral home had just come for my father's body, and I had just sat with Mother for a while. Mother was so withdrawn and showed no emotion, but that was okay. I cried a river for both of us. I tried to be a comfort for Mother but didn't know how she was feeling or what she was thinking. I just had to place myself back in time when she and Daddy had good health and remembered how much love they shared. I know they would have been devastated by the other's passing had their minds still functioned.

I remember that the drive out to my house was filled with tears. I collected myself long enough to call my dear friend Bretta and told her Daddy had passed. We sang him to heaven, and yet I felt so alone.

"Teresa," Bretta said softly, "of course you feel alone. When parents die, you naturally feel alone because they are gone, and you have become an orphan. They are no longer there to share their love with you."

O-r-p-h-a-n! Orphan. That is exactly how you feel, because you have never known a day of your life without them in it! Even though my mother was still with me physically, her mind was long gone. No feeling came from her. I did indeed become an *orphan* that day.

CHAPTER 12

Towers of Strength

As you go through life, you look around and you are surrounded by towers of strength. I have always been a people watcher. I find it interesting how people deal with different situations. I probably shouldn't, but we all tend to compare ourselves to how someone else handles stressful situations. You either compare how you have handled it or how you think you would.

I have two beautiful women from high school that I have always been good friends with. Best friends, as a matter of fact. But you know how life goes—distance, raising a family, just life getting in the way of being close.

> **"Would I ever get that peace in my heart ever again?"**

I would look at Bev in amazement at how she handled her mother dying at a young age and being an only child. I'm sure she was very sad, but she always had a smile on her face, and she seemed adjusted throughout the years.

Her father must have been an amazing man, keeping her focused and in normal situations. Her father has passed now and one of her sons. Those losses have taken a toll on her, yet she is still always smiling and seemingly in control. She is absolutely amazing.

My friend Susan is a different kind of amazing. Susan, like all of us do, watched her parents age. Susan was the older sister to a brother and sister. Her mother died when Susan was in her midforties. Susan helped her mother through cancer. Her father, a doctor, did so as well, and of course, he gave his wife particularly good care.

Susan stayed overnight with her mother for several days near the end. Susan recalls the final day and knew the processing out signs. She said she needed to run to a store to pick up a book and a few other supplies, and while she was gone, her mother passed. She said she felt like that was how her mother wanted to leave. She didn't want Susan to be there. Susan has peace in her heart about how it all went down that day.

Susan was then with her father in his years of going through AD. She did not have a relationship with her siblings like I had with mine. Hers was more strained.

Susan's father made some poor decisions in his later years, much to Susan's sadness and dismay, yet she seemed focused on helping as much as she could. His primary care was given by another sibling, which was hard on Susan because there were many things done that were out of her control. That in itself was very upsetting, and he did not receive the best care for someone with AD.

Susan was terribly angry at times. She knew in her heart this was a situation that she was simply going to have to let go of. She felt God had blessed her life with the best parents. She had a great life with them, and the care that was or was not given to her father was out of her control. She tried to give her opinions, but they fell on deaf ears.

She has wonderful memories, and no one can take those from her. She is very much at peace with the situation. She knows that others will answer to God for actions or non-actions. She still has that beautiful smile and peace in her heart.

Susan went with me to finalize the funeral arrangements for my parents. What a friend she was and seemed adjusted and in control. As I watched her sitting in that room with me, my thoughts were, *Would I ever get to that special place where the hurt is controlled and I can talk about them without a flood of tears or anger in my voice? Would I be able to remember my daddy and mother as they were when they were whole and healthy and fun-loving? These two friends had. Would I ever get that peace in my heart ever again?*

Another friend that I admire is Don. He lost his wife after several years fighting cancer. They were both in their forties—so young, with three children. Both were in their prime. She fought, and he fought with her. She was the love of his life, and they had married young. They didn't just love each other, but both felt like the sun rose and set in each other.

Don is a tower of strength, solid, but there were times when he felt weak and out of control. The horror of his love being destroyed, watching her before his eyes being taken over by the cancer and ripped from his heart was more than a human could bear. There were times, he said, that he was so mad—mad at the doctors, mad at God, mad at her and just plain mad, mad, mad!

Question after question came to him. Why and how could this happen? He was ashamed of being mad, and in the end your prayers change to wanting them to let go and be out of pain. Selfish feelings come out. You just want your life to be normal again, but you realize it will never be so.

On the outside, as I watched him, he always seemed in control. He was going on living, going about his work, raising a family and doing what a father does. Inside he was lost and just trying to make it. I could never tell from this side. What a tower of strength he displayed. My friend Steph went through watching her husband taken by cancer. Shortly after his death, his mother (her mother-in-law) passed as well. A few years later, Steph endured the passing of her daughter, also taken by cancer. Her daughter was only in her early fifties, leaving behind two children, one in high school and one in college. She suffered greatly, an agonizing ordeal for Steph to helplessly watch. A year after the torment of losing her daughter, Steph's aunt was stricken with AD.

Steph was a tower of strength, caring for each one, loving them through it all and falling to pieces inside every single time.

Steph remembers one time when she took her husband for treatment and wondered how she was going to get through another day. They were sitting in the waiting room, and Steph was silently praying. There was a woman sitting across from them with her husband, and they started a conversation. Steph, in her soft sweet voice, talked about what a tough day it was for them.

The woman said, "I know we all need the Lord, and He will see us through." With that, she asked if they could pray together and mentioned that she was the preacher at a nearby church.

Of course, Steph and Jim wanted to pray as well, so the four of them prayed together. As the woman led them, praying aloud, she started speaking in tongues. A calm suddenly came over both Jim and Steph. Steph said there was a very bright light in the room—so bright you couldn't see the walls. They knew at that very moment that God was with them, and He was in control and everything would be okay. It was amazingly powerful. Steph was reassured that she wasn't going through anything without God carrying her through.

Every Sunday evening, as we sat and played cards with these friends, there was always a conversation about our week. Our tears would flow. No one had answers. It was more of a vent session, a support group. It was therapy. Sharing our hearts and being able to vent, we realized that this is the progression of life. We live and we process out.

Our friends were there every step of my journey with my parents. It was a journey that was so heart-wrenching that at times it made no sense. There was no understanding of how two people who had lives that were so vibrant, energetic, youthful, dealing with the war, marrying, building a business and raising a family could reach a point of not knowing who they were or where they were. They did not know the names of their children or that the beautiful farm they were living on was the one they built. They no longer knew that the brush piles they burned, the thorn trees they cut down, the lake they developed, the land they mowed to look like a park all belonged to them.

Their minds could no longer comprehend anything around them. Physically, their bodies were strong, but their minds broke down in stages of decline. Their minds went back in time, back to youthful times. In his mind, Daddy was eighteen years old again, fighting the war over and over, telling the stories, going back there in his mind repeatedly and always telling the stories as if it were the first time.

Then he was sixteen again, playing basketball and farming for his mother and dad over and over again. Then he was back being twelve, having to get home. His mother and dad were waiting on him to come home. If he didn't get home, he would be in trouble; he had to get home. Then he regressed to about eight years old to four years old, then barely able to walk. Daddy had to be helped with a belt to hold him upright or with a wheelchair, and then the final stage was to be fed like an infant.

The family watched with disbelief at what was happening before their eyes. It was torture because nothing could be done. Some days they had clear minds, then in the blink of an eye, they were gone to years past.

As their daughter, I was frightened, I was scared, I was mad, I was saddened. I wanted to love, I wanted to hate, I wanted to run. The professionals will tell you that those feelings are a normal part of dealing with this disease, but they fail to tell you it can be all these different feelings felt within just a few seconds. You are reeling in the turmoil of it all, and you feel you are losing your own grip on reality.

I thank God for giving me many people around me, many towers of strength. I found myself thinking, *Okay, this person has gone through losing their parents, and they are still here, and they seem okay, so just maybe I'll make it through this.* "Towers of strength"—for without those people around me, I'm truly not sure how I would be here today.

CHAPTER 13

The Last Day

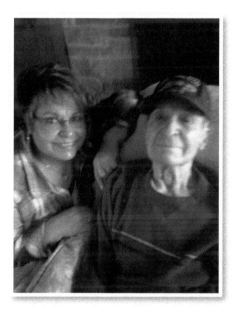

I was at Daddy and Mother's home one beautiful summer day. I worked around in the kitchen, cleaning up, wiping down the countertop, when Daddy said, "Teresa, come here." He was sitting in his wheelchair at the end of the table where he had just finished eating lunch. He sat there gazing out the window where they had a beautiful view that looked out over the backyard and flower bed of hollyhocks that grew there every year.

In that flower bed, Mother had an old red pump and a beautiful barn-shaped birdhouse feeder. You would see some beautiful birds and butterflies as you sat and looked out that window. Out past the barn and across the bean field to the fence line were pretty green trees, and sometimes deer or wild turkeys would be in the yard. It was a window to beauty, that was for sure. It was all so picturesque.

I walked over to him and said, "Yes, Daddy."

He looked up and said to me, "Thank you."

I said, "Daddy, why are you thanking me? What are you thanking me for?"

You must understand that someone with AD is not always there with you in their mind. They are gone somewhere in time, but at that moment, they are not here with you in the present. They will have a faraway look in their eyes. They do not know you or anyone.

This day was different. He said to me, "Well, just look!" With his hand, he motioned toward the window and said with a big smile, "Isn't it just beautiful?"

I said, "Yes, Daddy, it is! Would you like to go outside and sit on the patio for a while?"

"Yes!" was his immediate response.

I pushed him out onto the patio and got another chair and sat down next to him. I said, "Daddy, I'm trying my absolute best to keep this place going. As you can see, Stan has cut the hay, and it is baled."

In front and back of the house were fields of the big, round, one-ton hay bales. In Indiana, there really is just something about the smell of new-mown hay to us Hoosiers. When that smell is in the air, it does remind you of home. I'm sure that at that moment, he was thinking of home.

"We are keeping the grass mowed and the weeds cut," I told him. "Daddy, I know it isn't like how you kept it, but we sure are trying."

He said softly, "It is beautiful."

Then he turned to me and said, "I just can't quite figure out where my truck went."

"Daddy," I said, "a few months ago, you told me it was okay to sell it. We needed it out of the garage to make room for the handicap ramp we put in. I sold it to a young farmer, and it lives on a farm again, Daddy. I have the deposit slip to show you that I put the money in the bank."

He just waved his hand; he wasn't concerned about the money. He hollered for Mom and said, "Gracie, did you hear that? My truck is on a farm. I like that."

He turned to me and said, "This is the last day."

"Daddy, what do you mean?" I asked in a quavering voice.

My heart dropped, for I could not fathom what was next. I was enjoying having my father back. He was Dad, having a great conversation, playful and smiling. I was very scared of what I was going to hear next.

He leaned over to me and again said, "Thank you."

Then it was as if he were going to say something else…and at that very second, he drifted off in his own thoughts.

Remembering back to that day, I recall how I had hoped that somehow, some way, he would beat this horrible disease. I just had proof he could do this. He talked normally for a few minutes. He was Dad again! I knew, I just knew, that together, with my help, he would get through this!

But there is no coming back from AD. No, that was just wishful thinking on my part, not wanting to admit that we would not come out of this. What I realized was that it was his final goodbye to me. Yes, he lived about another year, but he kept declining. He would smile big when he heard my voice, but never again did we have a conversation about the present or really anything in the past. He knew he was in trouble. He knew this was not a great situation to be in, and that it was only going to get worse. And it did.

I realized that he loved me very much. He had the strength to come out for a few minutes, and it was especially important to him to tell me. My father was not good at saying "I love you" or "Goodbye." Never in my lifetime do I remember at the end of a phone conversation did he end it by saying, "Goodbye." It was always "Okay." *Click.*

However, he was wonderful at *showing* his love. I feel that day was for me. I felt special for that moment I had with my daddy. It gave me a small feeling of peace, but more emotions came over me, and I was saddened. I realized after that day that he was lost somewhere in time many years past, and I would never be able to reach him again. I truly feel that was the day Daddy departed.

CHAPTER 14

My Beautiful Daughter

Oftentimes, we look at our children who we have given birth to and we ponder, *Where did they come from? Why are* you *my child?* Sometimes they look like us and they act like us, but sometimes they are so amazing. You think, *No way did I create that human being!*

My daughter Amanda is one beautiful person. She is soft and tender, yet she is one of the strongest women I know.

I must go back a few years when she was very young, around twelve years old. She worked for me at my business, a cookie store in a mall. She was an excellent worker. Even though I was her mother, she could separate the mother/boss relationship. That is unusual for a young person to do; it showed great maturity. I always knew she would succeed in whatever she chose to do.

She has worked in the medical field for more than twenty years. She started out working in a rehab hospital for brain injury patients, right out of nursing school. She moved to the big city and has been there ever since. She has seen many life situations with patients and their families—some good, some bad, some happy and some just plain heartbreaking. She is one smart girl. Everyone speaks highly of her, and she is well liked and loved by many staff and patients.

Grandma and Grandpa were very proud of their granddaughter, and they loved her to the moon and back. Grandpa loved it that she loved to fish, and Grandma loved it that she was a nurse. My mother always thought a career in nursing would be wonderful. I feel Amanda was living Grandma's dream.

Amanda was one of my biggest supporters. She was there for me to bounce ideas off. She would let me vent when I was so mad and angry that this disease had taken my parents. If I did not understand medical terms, she explained them to me.

Amanda has always called me on her way home from work. Not every day, but she has not missed too many over the years. Some are short conversations, some have been long, some have been at a good time, some have been at a bad time. Yes, we have even gotten into some great conversations and some bad ones.

There was one in 2009 that was horrible and heartbreaking when she called. I had just been told that Daddy had AD, and I was still reeling from the news, trying to absorb what I had just been told minutes before. I know I started

> "No way did I create that human being!"

out denying, making excuses, expressing disbelief! Not my Daddy! This could not be! Then I had a sick feeling remembering moments, situations and gatherings when Daddy repeated his stories over and over. Thinking through those times, things came to mind, and I knew it was not a misdiagnosis. After much thought, I realized that it was spot on.

Amanda instantly heard in my voice that something was terribly wrong. I told her Daddy had AD. I could hear a silence on the other end, and then I heard her say, "I was afraid of that."

She kept it together for me at the time, asking questions about the medicines he was on and giving me ideas on how to help patients recognize family members. The nurse and the professional came out in her then. As I have said, she is incredibly good at what she does. After our conversation, I felt more positive and had a little better grip on what was ahead.

I never dreamed, though, that six years of decline would happen before my eyes. I couldn't foresee the coming debilitating changes. My daddy was a ball of fire, successful, owned and operated his own business and farm. He loved to fish, loved to tell stories, laugh and have fun. He never met a stranger, and most of all, he was the most positive person I have ever known. It could be dark gray and raining outside and he would tell you it was a beautiful day.

I remember one time, Daddy came back from the lake there on the farm. He had been cutting down thorn trees. There were many of them on the farm, and Mother was always saying how ugly those trees were.

Daddy just listened to her as Mother always had a way of emphasizing by her tone just how ugly she thought something was. He said, "Gracie, if we didn't have those old ugly trees, then we wouldn't know how beautiful the other ones are." Then he would always smile. Daddy always had a smile on his face.

Amanda was with me through several difficult situations and handled them beyond her years, and she helped me handle them better than I ever thought I could. We made a pretty awesome mother-daughter team. When parents or grandparents become ill (and I don't care what type of illness you are faced with), gather everyone around you—family, friends, caregivers, doctors, nurses, church family, anyone and everyone to help.

You cannot do it by yourself. It doesn't work; you will burn out. Share your experiences and listen to their tips. Every tip or suggestion will not work, but you don't know until you try. It does indeed take a village to help with the process, the decline. So build a team. Build a support team. Before it is finished, you will be amazed where support and help come from if you just open your mind and heart to the help. My beautiful daughter Amanda was there to help me build mine.

CHAPTER 15

Moving Day

I knew one day it would come to this, but somehow, someway, I was hoping it wouldn't be me to have to make that final decision to move them off the farm. I'm not sure, in my little girl thinking, who I thought was going to step up and do this horrible job requirement of being responsible. Yes, at times I wanted to be selfish. I wanted to break. I wanted my parents. I wanted to have a tantrum. God, I resented people who had their parents in good health.

> "Hold me, I was so afraid of the storm. I'll be safe in my Father's arms. Give God your storm. Put your hand in the hand of the man from Galilee. The Master is in control just like He was back then. Jesus already knows I'm going to make it through. Just keep trusting. We're in the same boat. There is nothing He won't bring you through. It has been quite a journey. God will be faithful."

Those are a few lines from songs by one of my favorite quartets that carried me through many storms with my parents, through the darkest days, the bleakest moments in my life. I could feel God guiding my steps through the words of those songs. He talked to me, and I would have moments of comfort and the turmoil would calm.

When I looked through my tears, many times I would see only one set of footprints. I knew He was holding and carrying me through this horrible part of life.

No matter how many times I listened to my favorite quartet, I have to admit it usually calmed me down by the time I made that thirty-mile drive to my parents' home. How it uplifted me, listening to those boys singing "We Believe," "You're Not Alone," "Put Your Hand in the Hand," "I Know My God Can,"

> "God, I resented people who had their parents in good health."

"It's Quite a Valley," "We're in the Same Boat," "Hold Me." It was God's way of helping me through. I sang at the top of my lungs and cried at the same time.

Somehow, I felt like it was God's way of talking to me. I felt the strain being lifted as He comforted me. Mentally, I felt myself easing down, going into almost neutral. It cleared my mind. He prepared me for the next round, the next stage. I felt in control by the time I reached Mother and Daddy's house. Sometimes I just sat in the car for a few minutes being still, quiet, and a calm would come over me. I knew God was there and He was with me. Once again, I thought, *Be still and know I'm God.*

The time approached to move them to a nursing home. Elizabeth and I had many conversations about the when and how this would proceed. She reported daily on every situation we had going on. Daddy was getting to where he could not walk to the bathroom or bed and was losing his balance totally. He had to be wheeled to the door, then two caregivers would lift him to the stool or bed, and Mother was the same way.

Mother fell in January and hit her head. It was downhill from that point. She went to the nursing home for a few weeks while we had the bathroom enlarged for the caregivers to shower Mother and Daddy, but she was also losing her balance and required two caregivers as well. The cost of home care was starting to escalate to astronomical heights. Four caregivers were needed around the clock.

As Mother and I had talked when we started on this journey, I had promised I would keep them on the farm in their home as long as they knew they were there. I'm sure you have heard it said to choose your words wisely. I was incredibly happy that I had chosen my words so carefully because if I had not, then the guilt would have been more astronomical for me than the cost.

We had reached expenses four times the cost of a nursing home with private home health care. We had the absolute best, and it was getting to be too much. It was starting to require more caregivers. Grant you, my parents were not poor, but on the other hand, they were not Bill Gates either. Everything they had worked for was going for their care. Me, my brother and sister all agreed it was their money and it went for their care. None of us had a problem with that.

Safety was very much a concern. We wanted them clean and well fed. They wanted for nothing. As we made the decision to move them to the nursing home, it tore my heart out. The team was tired, and it was costly to add more caregivers, so it was time. I started making arrangements. I wanted them near me, and the nursing home, of course, had to be the absolute best. After talking with several people, I found the one that was perfect for us. I made the agreement.

I brought in their lift chairs from home, blankets, TV, clothes and pictures to make their room as homey as I could. Everyone was impressed and complimented the decor. It was time to move them. This was the part that I wasn't sure I could do or even live through. Heart-wrenching? It goes beyond that. I knew this was never going to be good. They would not be returning to the place that had been their home for fifty years. I was taking that away from them.

The nursing home sent a van to pick them up. I was standing outside in the driveway, and Mr. Deb got out of the van. This man has the friendliest face any human has ever had. He asked me how I was doing, and with that, the tears flowed. I was sobbing.

He came over to me and said, "Oh, honey, it is okay. I'm here and I'm going to help you get through this. We will get through this, dear. I know it hurts, but sometimes we have to do what we have to do. This is all for the best. It doesn't seem like it right now, but it is."

After a few minutes, I started to calm down. Elizabeth wheeled Daddy out in his chair, and Sherry brought Mother out in hers. They were loaded into the van and ready to go.

Mr. Deb gave me a big hug and said, "It will be okay. Just follow me to the nursing home and we will do this together."

Down the hill we went, down that long lane, and of course I was bawling and crying out, "Lord, have mercy! What have I done? Please, Mommy and Daddy, don't hate me! Please, Lord, what have I done?"

I was trying to get hold of my husband. His phone went to voice mail, or so I thought. I was so distraught. I needed someone to tell me, "You're okay and they will be okay."

That's exactly what my husband, Joe, was telling me, but I didn't hear him. I was incoherent. Joe was so upset hearing me saying those pleas to God and was trying to calm me down, and I hung up on him!

At that point, I was nearing the end of the lane. The storm inside my head swirled with scenes of precious memories: me getting off the bus and walking up that long lane, Mother being home waiting with her smile, the smell of her cooking dinner and her asking how my day was at school. Memories of Daddy getting home from work and helping me with my horse, me driving my brother's green VW bug down to the end of the lane to get the mail. What fun! (Of course, that was a big deal since I was only twelve years old!)

Not too many years ago, Daddy, at the age of eighty, was jogging every day from the house down to the end of the lane to get the mail. All these thoughts and memories ricocheted around in my head. I was nearing the end of a different time, my life, their life. I felt helpless! I was ending their time there.

I reached the end of the lane and was ready to pull onto the road, and I looked through my tears. All I could see was the backs of their heads as they sat together in their wheelchairs, side by side. That was how it had been for them for sixty-eight years of marriage, side by side. They both appeared sound asleep with their heads bowed down together. They never even knew they left the farm. They truly had already left at a much earlier time. Thank you, dear Jesus. Thank you!

CHAPTER 16

The Nursing Home

When we arrived at the nursing home, the staff was a little confused with the two caregivers we kept on the payroll until my parents' passing. Why were they there? I felt that Mother and Daddy had seen Elizabeth and Jenny for a couple of years, and I didn't want to confuse them with all the new people around them. I wanted them to feel secure and see familiar faces.

I explained my thinking and that it had nothing to do with Jenny or Elizabeth telling the nursing home staff how to do their jobs. It was strictly for Mr. and Mrs. Williams' comfort. As their daughter, I would be the one to tell them how I wanted the job done. I think they finally understood that I did expect things to be done correctly and in a timely manner, and I did get their respect.

Of course, food does help as a great persuader. When I found out that one of the nurses had a birthday or "just because," then pizza, cookies, doughnuts, candy and cake would show up. It all helps to show your appreciation for their willingness to be part of a team.

We did have one problem, but it was corrected. When the house cleaning crew came in to clean, they got hot from their strenuous efforts. They turned the air-conditioning down to sixty-eight degrees, and then they left and did not turn it back up. Mother would get cold, and her hands and feet were like ice cubes when I came in.

She did not talk much and couldn't walk to the closet to get a sweater or a blanket, and she was unable to get to the air conditioner to reset it. Needless to say, I was upset because she had been cold for quite a while. All this was unnecessary suffering, all because of thoughtless people. I would turn the air-conditioning back up.

The first time I brought it to the staff's attention, I politely asked if they could please say something to the crew. The second time, I hung a sign on the air conditioner, requesting to please remember to adjust the temp back to

> "Of course, food does help as a great persuader."

seventy-eight degrees. Then I came in and the sign was gone, and the air was still at sixty-eight degrees. Well, let me tell you, the third time with me and "You're *out!*" The third time I will tell you how it will be done, and I did.

I asked for a meeting with the floor manager, nurse supervisor and nursing home director to get to the bottom of this problem. I was happy to inform them what my course of action would be. I explained that I had asked twice for this to be addressed, and it was not corrected. So I laid out my plan of action.

"This is what I will do, and you can be assured this is how I will proceed to correct this problem. I'm just giving you a heads-up!" I told them. "The air conditioner in my parents' room, which I pay $11,500 for each month, will be set to my specifications. The next time I come in and find that it is not, I will cut the cord off of it, and we won't worry about those that can't keep their hands off it. We will no longer have an issue!"

After that, Mother was always warm, the problem was solved and I'm fairly sure we understood each other from that point on. We never had a problem again.

CHAPTER 17

Labor Day and a Labor of Love

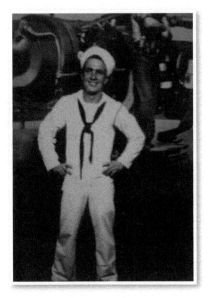

Labor Day weekend started out like any other Labor Day. We owned a business, and this was an extremely busy weekend for our sporting goods store. Summer was winding down. Boating, camping and picnics were ending. The summertime fun was over, and kids were heading back to school. I had stopped by on Sunday morning to check on Mother and Daddy on my way into the store. As always, I walked into their room, and Daddy was sitting up in his lift chair. He had a big smile on his face.

"Hi, Daddy!" I greeted him, and for about five seconds, the lost look was gone.

He said, "Hi, honey!" And with that, he was gone again.

I said, "How are you today, Daddy?"

The faraway look crossed his face, and he didn't speak again. He just had that big smile on his face. Mother hadn't been attended to yet and was still in her bed. She half smiled. I gave her and Daddy a doughnut and some coffee, and it was time for Mother's shower. I told them goodbye and gave each a hug, and I went to work.

Again, about noon, I ran out to see them, and they had been taken to lunch. Sunday, the weekend of Labor Day, is our slow time for the holiday weekend. It's over, and everyone is getting ready to leave and are going home from the park. I decided to head home and get ready for our little picnic that we had planned with friends and family. Joe had closed early, and off we went to our picnic. About an hour into it, the nursing home staff called and told me Dad's breathing was very labored, that he was shutting down and they had called in hospice.

Of course, Joe and I went right back into the nursing home. When we got there, they told us to prepare for Daddy's processing out. They suggested that we make phone calls to anyone we thought he would like to hear from and hold the phone to his ear, letting them talk to him while he listened. The nurse explained that hearing is the last of the senses to go.

With that, I called my daughter, and they came from Indianapolis as quickly as they could. We continued to talk to Daddy all evening, and we sang him to heaven with many different songs, songs he loved. We read verses out of the Bible. We told stories. At about 11:00 p.m., Amanda went out to our house to get some sleep. I promised her that if anything got worse, I would call her in.

The nurses made Daddy as comfortable as possible in that situation. They came in about every four hours with a shot. During that time, we kept checking on Mother as she was in bed on the other side of the room from Daddy. In the room, only their lift chairs separated them. Mother was comfortable but seemed very scared as this situation kept unfolding. I was trying to keep her informed, but I wasn't sure what to do.

It was Monday, Labor Day, around 5:00 a.m. Joe nor I had really slept. We had just dozed now and then. For some reason, both of us had fallen asleep, and all of a sudden, over my nose floated a sweet, fruity smell. I looked around, and nothing had been sprayed in the room. Very puzzled, I got up and I looked in the bathroom. Mother cannot walk or go by herself. I thought maybe someone had come in and placed some kind of deodorizer in the bathroom. I went to the hallway thinking that maybe the cleaning crew had started in cleaning, but everyone was very quiet. Still the smell hovered around my nose.

I walked back to the chair beside my Daddy, and I held his hand and started crying because I realized what the fragrance was. It was Juicy Fruit gum. When I was a little girl, Daddy and Mother owned their own business. When they ordered something for the business, they would have to go pick it up at the bus station, and that was me and Daddy time.

I was about four years old, and he would holler, "Come on, we have to go to the bus station!" It was a fun ride downtown, and he would buy packs of Juicy Fruit gum for him and one for me. Daddy would have his chewed up by the time we would return to the store. I, on the other hand, would chew only one or two pieces. I loved going. We always had fun, and I loved the smell of that gum. Something so simple brings back those precious memories.

I truly think that Daddy was getting my attention and letting me know that everything was okay. As morning approached, my daughter came back in. I called my brother, and he talked to Dad for a while on the phone. My sister came in and said her goodbyes. I called my son Blaine who lived in Okinawa, Japan, at that time, and he talked to Grandpa and said his goodbyes. I called his sisters in, and they sat with Daddy until he passed. They helped sing him to heaven, too, along with the pastor from hospice. She was a beautiful woman, and she had a beautiful singing voice, a voice like an angel.

My daughter, even though she is Grandpa's granddaughter, is a nurse as well. She was with me every step, and she let me know when it was time for the last shot. She is a beautiful soul, and she has the biggest brown eyes and the most beautiful full lips and skin like a china doll. Watching her sing to her grandpa and the way she talked to him softly and very lovingly, it made me proud she was my daughter and my daddy's granddaughter. When she looked over at me with tears in her eyes and mouthed "last one," I just shook my head. Yes, and my eyes filled with tears as well.

She reached over suddenly and said to Grandpa as she was getting his hat off the nightstand and placing it on his head, "Grandpa, you have your hat on now. I love you, Grandpa. You can go now that you have your hat."

With that, Daddy did go. It was only a couple of minutes until he took his last breath. I know it sounds silly, but he loved that hat, and he was so proud of that hat. His grandson Blaine was in the invasion of Iraq. When Blaine was returning from war, we met him in Hawaii, and Daddy, Grandpa, was allowed to ride on the ship, the *Duluth*, with Blaine back to California. That was a huge deal! Daddy was so proud and so proud of his grandson.

It was Dad's *Duluth* hat that Amanda put on his head—the one Blaine had given him as a remembrance of their time together. Daddy had worn that hat ever since. I'm sure it brought back many memories of the ship he was on in World War II, the *LST-647*. Daddy served with the amphibian forces of the United States Navy in the pre-invasion of Okinawa. He was a pointer on one of the twin 40mm guns. He also served in combat in the invasion of Okinawa and Ie Shima where they landed infantry, amphibian tanks and Ernie Pyle, our war correspondent.

The *LST-647* had been on a considerable adventure just before L-Day. It steamed around Okinawa twice to confuse the enemy about their intentions. It then broke off to the southeast and the island named Kerama Retto. The night they circled Okinawa, *LST-647* was called to battle stations eight times.

As the *LST-647* and the other ships they traveled with entered the bay. They discovered 119 Japanese patrol boats. These patrol boats were fast, powered by large Chrysler engines, and were capable of making speeds up to sixty miles per hour. Most were rigged with high explosives which could detonate on collision with another boat. They were suicide boats designed to attack the American fleet when it came for the invasion of Okinawa.

Immediately when discovering the suicide boats, the *LST-647* called for air support from a nearby aircraft carrier. Within minutes, the Hellcats arrived and set upon the 119 suicide boats. As my Daddy watched from the gun tub, one suicide boat moving extremely fast was passing right by him. It escaped, then it re-entered the harbor where it shared the fate of the other suicide boats.

The *LST-647's* discovery of the 119 suicide boats before they fired had been a big save for the fleet. Daddy could definitely relate to the men that had just gone through the invasion in Iraq. Daddy was always proud of the service he gave, and he was immensely proud of his grandson as well.

CHAPTER 18

Rebecca, My Cousin but More Like a Sister

I never called her Rebecca. I called her Becky. Through my life, she has been my buddy. We have always been close, and as life would have it, we both married our high school sweethearts. These men were completely different in their own right. They were so different from the men we are married to today. We both look at each other, puzzled as to why. Both of us do know one thing: we are very blessed with the children we have and know that the creation of those children was the reason for those marriages.

Because of being busy raising families, moving because of jobs, living in different locations, our closeness has been strained at times. From 1960 to 1980, communication was not what it is today with Facebook, e-mails, and cell phones. It was snail mail at best, and who had time to write when you were in the middle of raising children?

> **"It was always a fun day when we played for hours out there under those trees."**

Nonetheless, we remained close even with different crises in our lives, with divorce, children marrying, deaths. When we were growing up, they were the Sunday afternoon relatives that came, or we went to their house. Becky's mother (my aunt Middy) and my mother were sisters. My aunt Middy made the best pie and fried chicken ever made. No one could hold a candle to her cooking.

There were four years between my cousin Becky and me. Now that we are old women, that is not so much a big deal, but growing up, it was a *very* big deal! When she was twelve years old, I was only eight. I still loved dolls, but let me tell you a secret. She did too! We played house. I remember one of the best times was being at our grandparents' home in their front side yard where they had small sapling-type trees.

We played for hours, pretending that those trees were our mansion with many different rooms. We dressed up in grandma's old mismatched high-heeled shoes and carried her big black umbrella around, acting like we were very rich with countless servants. Of course, we had our baby dolls, so we had many children. We were hostesses for an afternoon imaginary tea party that was enjoyed by all our imaginary friends.

It was always a fun day when we played for hours out there under those trees. Both of us were sad when it was time to go. I can only wonder, had it been more like today with all the technology, how close we would have been and how life would have gone so many different directions. Maybe in our case, it was best that it was the time it was. It gave us many precious memories.

As I mentioned before, Aunt Middy was my mother's sister, and our families were very close. Summertime meant picnics, boating and fishing. Wintertime meant get-togethers, dinners, card games for the adults and board games for the kids.

Becky's dad, my uncle Francis (I called him Uncle Fritz), was an unusual man. He served in the Army in WWII. But he was different from my father because he worked for the Pfizer Company. My aunt never drove a car, though I'm not sure why. I know they had a terrible car accident. She went through the windshield of the car, and she just never had an interest in driving after that.

Uncle Fritz was good to her, and he took her and the kids to town every Saturday for her to shop, and it worked for them. He retired from Pfizer. He enjoyed golf, bowling and camping. They enjoyed many travels and were Snowbirds in Florida during the winter. One thing about my Uncle Fritz, he loved to talk.

Daddy, on the other hand, left Pfizer after ten years and went into business for himself. He sold a farm, bought another one, built a new home, had cattle and horses. Mother worked alongside my dad as she was the accountant for the company. She was very independent and drove everywhere. Daddy didn't play golf or bowl, but he did love to fish, rabbit and bird hunt, go boating and eat fried chicken.

What the two men had in common was this: both men loved their wives and families and enjoyed life, but most of all they loved to talk. I'm not sure who could out-talk who, and I'm not sure who told the biggest fish tales. Uncle Fritz thought Benny was "a fart in a whirlwind," and my Daddy would say, "Oh, that Fran-cee, he's something!" and just laugh! Both couples had a particularly good relationship through the years and were remarkably close.

As the years went by and my father showed signs of AD, it was heartbreaking for my Uncle Fritz. He would fish Daddy's lake and enjoyed going by and talking with Dad. Mother and Dad would always invite him in for a cup of coffee, and Daddy always offered up graham crackers. Daddy always said you just had to have a good cup of coffee and a cracker of some kind to make the fishing better. Knowing Dad, he just meant that good conversation was what it was all about.

That all happened less and less as Daddy showed more and more visible signs that something was wrong. Uncle Fritz was older and in fairly good shape. It was simply hard for him to accept that times were changing. He was like all of us, thinking that Daddy was supposed to live forever. This should not be happening. It just made Uncle Fritz angry, and I don't think my uncle could get past the anger.

Becky and I would talk often about the changes we were seeing in both men. Her mother had died of lung cancer and heart problems fairly suddenly. We were watching our parents as they were aging. We had many discussions, but of course, as I have said many times throughout the chapters in this book, discussions were about the extent of it. There were no plans or actions.

Attempting to help or expressing our opinion with them was at times impossible. Often it was not heard. Maybe they heard us, but they wouldn't accept what we were trying to tell them. They were "The Greatest Generation." We knew without a doubt in our minds that they would go down doing it their way.

Uncle Fritz was in his nineties, was in love with a little waitress at a local eatery, lived by himself, grew a beard and mustache that was snow white and wore a fedora. He carried a cane, drove a white convertible and looked like Colonel Sanders. There were times when people would comment about him looking like or ask if he was Colonel Sanders. He loved the notoriety.

As time will take a toll on the aging, Uncle Fritz was not immune. He was getting a little weaker a few months at a time, with just the aging process, things wearing out and the processing out. At one point, he had fallen, and the doctor suggested he do rehab for a few weeks. So with the doctor's recommendation, he entered an assisted living facility and started his rehab.

Becky came to see my dad, her Uncle Benny, not knowing when she walked into the nursing home that Uncle Benny had passed away about twenty minutes earlier. Everything was a little chaotic, and she gave me a hug and told me how much she loved me and that it would be okay. She was on her way to see her own dad. She said they were going to get something to eat and go see him. Through our tears, we hugged, and she was on her way.

As they travelled there (twenty-eight miles away), she got a call from her sister-in-law, saying, "Dad is gone."

Becky said, "Linda, did he check himself out? Did he go home? He has done this before. He gets to thinking he doesn't need rehab, that his leg will get better, it will heal, he doesn't need these exercises. Go check at the house and see if he is there. We will be there shortly."

Linda paused and said, "No, Beck. He is gone. He just passed away."

Of course, Becky was caught totally off guard. She was having trouble wrapping her head around this. He was fine the day before. He had even called her during the night at about 1:00 a.m. He wanted to make sure she would bring him clean clothes in the morning because he didn't have any for when it was time to go home. She assured him that she would.

That was the last time she talked to him, and he had seemed perfectly fine. When she got there, she was given the time of his passing, and in her heart, she couldn't help but smile. When she called to tell me the news, my phone went to voice mail, and she left the message for me that said, "Daddy and Uncle Benny have gone fishing. They died about forty minutes apart. They were the best of buddies, good fishing buddies, had great times through the years and they are going to continue to have good times. I'm sure Mother had fried chicken ready for them when they got there."

My heart was sad. Yet if you knew how it had been through the years with dinners, vacations together, lots of good times and many, many precious memories, then you couldn't help but smile and know they wouldn't have done it any other way.

CHAPTER 19

Pink Easter Egg

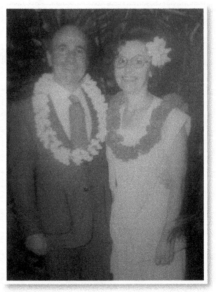

Our son is a military man with twenty-two years in the Marine Corps. Needless to say, we are all extremely proud of him. He is serving our country well. He has had thirteen tours in Iraq and Afghanistan and countries I don't even know where and most of the time can't even pronounce. Being in Special Forces, he has done other tours we know nothing about, and it is probably best we do not know.

The girls, his siblings, love their brother, but they also think he is the special one, "angel baby," and that angels sing when he enters a room. (They all four mimic an angel chorus when he does, and we all laugh!) They love to tease me about him, and it is all in fun.

Like any parent or grandparent, all our children are special in their own way. Children reflect traits and habits of each parent, and when you see yourself in them, of course you love seeing that, and it is special. It never makes one child or grandchild more important than another. My daddy and mother had nine grandchildren, and I know they were immensely proud of each and every one of them.

My sister's boys are in farming, and one of them sold honey, eggs and garden vegetables all through school, beginning when he was quite young. When he was about twenty years old, he bought a new John Deer combine straight from the factory. He is a very accomplished young man and farms thousands of acres of land. His brother, a Purdue graduate, owns his own business, and his beautiful wife is a professor at the local college. They are a remarkable family. It is just interesting to see many differences in each one.

My brother's three boys are brilliant like my brother, all college men. All of them hold fantastic jobs. One of them, Sam, is in the Coast Guard. He graduated from the Academy. I'm sure the position admiral is in his future.

My daddy served in World War II in the Navy, and he loved hearing about Blaine's achievements in the Marine Corps. The Bronze Star with Valor is among a few of Blaine's awards, and that was about the last one that Dad could comprehend. Blaine's relationship with Grandpa went back to when he was a little boy. He loved listening to Grandpa tell war stories, and Daddy had many stories to tell.

A man wrote a book about Ernie Pyle and came to Dad's home early in the 2000s and interviewed him several times. Dad had many stories about Ernie Pyle. Dad was with Mr. Pyle the day before he was killed. He told about the conversations they had that day. Dad was also at the invasion of Ie Shima and the invasion of Okinawa, Japan. I also know the History Channel came and interviewed Dad as well. It was pretty awesome seeing your dad on TV relating his war stories for the world to hear.

My children and I had a ritual every Veteran's Day. I would take the kids out of school for the day, and we went to Grandpa's house and listened to his war stories. Blaine loved listening to his Grandpa.

Blaine and his family were stationed on Okinawa at the time of Dad's passing. It was the Labor Day holiday when Dad passed. I had notified the family that Dad was passing. Some came, and some called. I had a conversation with Blaine and held the phone to Grandpa's ear so Blaine could tell his Grandpa how much he loved him.

Those are the moments that are heart-wrenching. When I returned the phone to my ear, all Blaine could utter was, "Love you, Mom," and I responded the same. We hung up. It was late night in Japan. We both knew when we hung up that the next phone call would be at the time of Dad's death, and neither one of us looked forward to that.

Blaine said his sleep was terrible that night and he awoke out of a restless sleep and got up much earlier than usual, still dark out. He decided to walk his big German shepherd. Gunner is a big boy. I always told Blaine I wasn't sure who was walking who. Even though it was earlier than he usually walked, Blaine thought the fresh air would help him.

As he walked, he had the feeling that Grandpa had passed even though he had not received verification from me. It was just a feeling he had. He said he felt his Grandpa's presence with him. Blaine said he was thinking of World War II and Okinawa. Then he wondered if he would receive a sign from Grandpa.

Blaine said that there was a huge church building in the middle of the area where he walked. It takes a few minutes for him to pass around the building to get back to his home. He looked at one of the windows of the church, and it has many windows. In one of them, a light was going off and on.

Blaine thought it was very strange because all the other windows in the church were dark, no lights on anywhere. There was no movement, no cars parked anywhere in any of the parking lots, but there was a light flickering in one window.

Blaine said he thought, *Okay, Grandpa, you have my attention.* As he walked on, suddenly, he looked down and there, sitting on the sidewalk in the middle of nothing else, was a pink Easter egg. There were no other Easter eggs, toys of any kind or litter. Remember, this was Labor Day, in September!

Blaine bent over and picked up the pink egg. He said out loud, "That is pretty funny, Grandpa. You drove off on Easter a few years back, and you know I was trying to help Mom not be so upset and stressed. I made a joke about you driving off. When we were kids, you always hid the Easter eggs, and that year you decided to hide yourself instead of the eggs.

"Mom cried and she laughed when I made that joke," he continued, talking aloud in the darkness. "I knew in my heart, Grandpa, that you would think that was pretty funny. Mom said when she told you what I had said, you laughed and giggled, thinking it was really funny. Love you, Grandpa. Thanks for the reminder of fun times and laughter we shared over the years. Fly high, Grandpa, fly high!"

Blaine held a ceremony on base, honoring his Grandpa. He has kept the pink Easter egg in a glass box. Grandpa and Blaine shared an incredibly special relationship, one that Blaine will always cherish.

CHAPTER 20

October With Mother

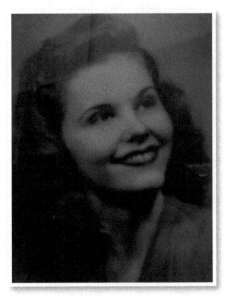

Fall in Indiana is usually beautiful. The trees are turning colors, bright yellows, reds, greens and amber. The smell of burning leaves, leaves dropping and the covered bridge festival all mark this season. It was my mother's favorite time of year. Just cool enough that a sweater would be all you needed to wear with jeans and boots. No heavy coats or gloves were necessary.

She loved being outdoors and raking leaves. The farm had many trees, and it was beautiful in the fall. The house was set back a lane in a wonderful setting, and it really was most gorgeous in the fall. It came as no surprise to me that Mother would pass at this time of the year.

I felt Mother had hung on for Daddy. She knew Daddy had AD, and she did her very best to take care of him, and she did. She covered for him when he had really slipped in his behavior and his hygiene. Love is everything, and she protected him. She said one time that she loved everything that started with the letter *B*: bread, baskets, babies, butterflies, birdies, bunnies and her Benny. That was Daddy's name.

I guess she was afraid if we had known the situation they were in, we would exercise our voice and demand that caregivers come in to help or send them to a nursing home. She had problems of her own. Dementia had set in and was taking a toll on her. She fought the best fight until she couldn't hide it anymore, and it was out of control.

After Daddy passed, I knew in my heart she wouldn't be with us much longer without him. Every day I would go by and see her two or three times a day. I tried to take her something to drink or ice cream, and I would push her wheelchair outside every day to brighten her day. She was asleep 90 percent of the time. I knew she had totally given up. She no longer wanted to live without Daddy. She had not talked much in the last six months, but in the last twenty-eight days after Daddy passed, she never said another word. Maybe she would force a faint smile.

I would read to her. I had a bird book that you could push a button and the pictured bird would sing or whistle. She loved that book! She would hear the birds and would look around as if the bird were right there in her room, and I would ask her what kind of bird it was. Then I would read the descriptions of the birds. You could tell she really enjoyed that book.

I would also read a devotional every day. She also seemed to enjoy the *Chicken Soup* series of books. The nursing home staff called me early one morning to tell me that Mother was having trouble breathing, and they had called hospice. I knew when they called hospice that she didn't have long to live.

I called my daughter Amanda. I have no idea how I could have gotten through any of this without my daughter and my husband. They both were my support and my rocks, keeping me anchored.

We sat with Mother until the end and played some of her favorite songs. We sang her to heaven just as we did Daddy. Some of her favorite songs included "The Old Rugged Cross," "Mansion over the Hilltop," "In the Garden," and "Amazing Grace." I read some of her favorite Bible verses: John 3:16, Psalms 23, and Ecclesiastes, a season for everything.

When I was a little girl, Mother would lie down with me in the afternoon for a nap. Sometimes it is hard to get a small child to be still, but Mother had a way of settling me down. She would read a story in a very soft voice and rub my arm and tell me she loved me. Mother had such soft, gentle hands.

As a little girl, I usually had long hair, and Mother would brush and comb my hair. It was a routine on Saturday evenings to clean up for Sunday church. All week, you had baths, but somehow this was different. It was like a beauty shop experience for me. Mother washed my hair and curled it with those pink sponge curlers.

She even gave me permanents because my hair was very straight, and she thought curls were a very nice change. She was gentle, and I loved the attention. Somehow, she always made me feel special and very loved. Those hands were so soft and gentle.

That day, as we were preparing for her to pass, I laid my head on the bed beside her, and my arm was against her side, and she started rubbing my arm. I knew at that precise moment she was telling me it was okay. She knew who I was and that she loved me. I held her as she took her last breath, and my heart shattered.

Many emotions flooded my soul. Mother hated the dark, and as I was holding her, I prayed that she was flying like a beautiful butterfly, that it was a bright and beautiful journey, and that Daddy was waiting on his Gracie. I thanked God that He had given me such a beautiful mother, and I know in my heart I will see her again someday.

CHAPTER 21

A Visitation and a Realization

I have often read that writing out your thoughts and feelings help you deal with your emotions. The way I feel right now, this very minute, I know for sure there are not enough pages in this little book.

It has been one week since the sale, the auction. By definition, *auction* is a public sale where goods or property is sold. That doesn't even come close to what an auction is.

It is an event where pieces of your heart are ripped away and sold to the highest bidder. It is an ending to part of your life as you remembered it, precious memories from years ago. Those pieces of things, stuff, antiques, junk are meaningless to the auctioneer and the buyers. Only the one who owns those treasures knows their meaning. These things took a lifetime to build and only a few hours to deplete.

All week building up to the sale, I was torn if I had made the right decisions. I was worried. My mother and daddy enjoyed their farm and their antiques. They enjoyed the hunt, the quest, the adventure of the find. They loved taking something old and making it beautiful. It was never about selling it and making money from it. It was truly about the collection.

My daddy built a red brick building to house those treasures, to house a collection of antiques and seventeen antique carriages. Each carriage was museum quality. The Amish in Arthur, Illinois, rebuilt and refinished each and every one. There was a single-seat doctor's carriage, a lady's carriage, Big Red (a carriage with fringe on top), just to name a few. The most beautiful of all was the Big Coach. I always loved it. It reminded me of a Cinderella carriage.

That buggy shed, as Daddy called it, or the carriage house, as my Mother called it, was a museum, and every item in it was museum quality. What I found to be so interesting was that every time you walked into that building, you noticed something different as you looked around at the antiques hanging in the rafters and on the walls.

There were hammers, crocks, steel traps, telephone pole insulators, screen doors, baby carriages, an apple press, antique carriage tools, cabinets, beer signs—the list is long and goes on and on. It seemed as if something new, something you had never seen before, would appear, and when you would ask Dad about it, he would say, "Aw, that has been there for a long time." It was such an interesting and fun place.

> "It is an ending to part of your life as you remembered it, precious memories from years ago."

My heart broke as I was now selling it piece by piece. I hired the best auctioneer and team that money could buy. We advertised and spared no money promoting it. Even our local TV station picked up on the story and ran reports about the up-and-coming auction several times in a two-day period. (You can't even buy that kind of advertising!) With all that said, I felt like I was destroying a lifetime of memories.

I started out Friday at the farm with a preview of the auction. It was open to the public, and people from around the county and from all over the state came and looked. My stomach was in a knot, and I was starting to panic. I said to our auctioneer, Jeff, "Can we pull the plug on this? I'm not sure I can go through with it. I will pay you your hours and whatever percent you need."

Jeff just kind of stood for a minute and then said, "Teresa, do you think that would be the right thing to do?"

I had tears in my eyes, and I said, "No, it is just so hard."

He said, "I know it is. It is never easy for the family."

I have to say that Jeff Boston and his wife, Amy, are wonderful people. They are the kindest, most gentle souls that you could ever meet. God used them as tools for His work. They were so kind and helped me through this sale of precious memories. I'm not sure I would have made it through without their guidance and expertise.

A dark-haired lady and her husband from New Jersey came up the drive near the end of the preview. She wanted to look around and expressed interest in the house. She really wasn't interested in the carriages and other antiques, though she did make a remark that she thought everything was so nice. We walked in the house. She looked around, and she turned to me and said, "I bet you had fun growing up here!"

I said, "Yes, I did. It was pretty awesome. I had horses, and I just loved it!"

She said, "I know."

I looked at her, and she just smiled at me.

She walked around the house just looking and touching the walls and cabinets, not really saying a whole lot. We walked back outside, and she said to me, "You have a lake."

It was not really a question, more like a statement. I was a little puzzled as to how she knew and it was okay, yet I felt somewhat odd. I asked her if she would like to see it, and I told her we could drive back to it. When we got back to the lake, we walked through the campsite that we had there next to the lake. She stood and turned to me and said, "Your mommy and daddy are here!"

I was quite surprised but felt calm as we walked back to her car. Once there, she turned to me and said, "Your mommy and daddy are very proud of you."

I have to say, of all the things that I needed that day, with all the emotions that were churning inside me, that's what I needed to hear most of all—that my parents were proud of me!

As the next day arrived and we were waiting for carriages to sell, I felt sick to my stomach. I went behind our old Ford truck and vomited a couple of times, trying very hard to keep my wits about me and trying very hard to stay calm and in control. Item by item was selling and leaving. People were everywhere, looking over things. An old family friend and his wife were buying items. They bought the old yellow veggie wagon, and they were smiling from ear to ear, so proud that they had gotten it.

At that very moment, it came to me. *I'm not destroying these things of Daddy and Mother's. They will live on and on, maybe not on the farm in the red brick building, but each item will live on in many places and will be enjoyed by many.*

As I was in a conversation with a man whom I worked with for many years, I happened to look over at the double glass door at the back of the house. There stood the dark-haired lady from New Jersey. Wearing sunglasses, she was standing by the big tree, and she spotted me and gave me a big smile. She held her hand up under her chin and gave me a little wave.

I was stunned. My mother had waved like that many times throughout my life. I was a cheerleader all through school, and when I was at games out on the floor cheering, she would be up in the bleachers, and we would smile at each other and do our little wave.

When I showed horses out in the arena, she would spot me in the lineup and do that little under-the-chin wave. I always knew she was there, and she was my biggest fan and supporter. I always knew I was never alone. That day was no different, for I knew I had been sent a reminder that she was there with me and I was not alone.

CHAPTER 22

I'm Gittin' Married

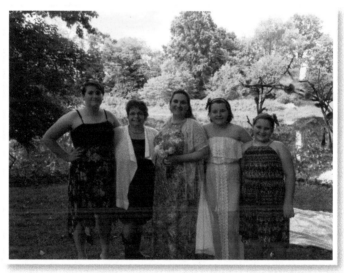

My mother and I loved to sing together. Mother loved Ann Murray, and in the evening, she would put her album on, and we would belt out a few of her songs. Not sure we ever did it justice, but we would sing one we loved and that Daddy loved: "Could I Have This Dance?" Daddy would lay on the floor and listen to us sing.

Another singer my Daddy loved to listen to was his little sister, my aunt Mary. He drove her to Nashville, Tennessee, a couple of times to sing on the Grand Ole Opry. She cut a record, and one of her songs was "'I'm Gittin' Married."

This song came to mind when our daughter announced she was getting married again. We sort of felt like it was nearing because when you would see the two of them together, you just knew there was a fire between them. She was finally marrying her high school sweetheart. They had gone different ways, and their lives drifted apart, but one class reunion brought them together again. He was wonderful with her three girls.

Mother absolutely loved Bob, and when he walked in the room, she would light up and her eyes were on him. One would think he walked on water. The way she smiled, there was no doubt in anyone's mind that she thought he was something.

Our daughter thought the weekend of the carriage sale would be a very stressful weekend for me, but maybe if we also had something to look forward to like her wedding, maybe it would help it to be less stressful. At first, she hated to say anything about it, but she said the more she thought about it, it was what her mother needed.

She asked my opinion, and at first, I wasn't sure, but the more I thought about it, I felt she had the right idea. No doubt in my mind that was one of the worst times in my life dealing with the sale, but knowing that the next day family and friends would be gathered around our daughter and her new husband was a good focus and a good distraction.

We were busy setting up for the wedding down by her favorite spot on the farm, the fishing hole. She fished there with her grandpa many times. Many memories were made on that farm, and she wanted to feel that her grandpa and grandma were there with her that special day. I, too, wanted her to feel them there.

I had this idea that for a very special gift, I would sing "Could I Have This Dance?" I worked hard on the song, sang it many times, practicing for my husband. He thought it sounded great. When working with the band, they knew how hard it was for me. Most of the time, I couldn't get through it without crying, but I was determined to get through it for her.

The boys would always sing through it and never miss a beat. The big day came. I felt I had my calm about me and could get through it.

Not even close. Everything flooded through me like a hurricane: the death, the farm, the sale. Our beautiful daughter was getting married to a new man, not only in her life and her daughters' but ours as well.

It was a new start in all our lives. Celebrating without my daddy and mother there on their farm was unfamiliar to all of us. The tears flowed down my cheeks, and I couldn't give her the gift. The band was great, and they carried on for me. It was too much for me.

I wasn't the only one who had problems carrying on. Amanda and Bob had asked my husband, Papa Joe, to marry them. There was no problem with that as he was licensed. All papers were signed, and at the end of the ceremony, when he blessed them, he introduced them as Mr. and Mrs. Holmes, not Hines.

It goes to show that stress does a lot of things to people. Everyone there were family and friends, and everyone understood what a tough time all of us were having. They were all so supportive and comforting through it all. Your family and friends need to be cherished because it is all over before you know it.

CHAPTER 23

Not Just a Bowl

Precious memories abound when you have to dispose of your parents' household items. It is a most difficult task, no matter their age or the cause of their passing. Some items you just can't part with. Usually they are not big expensive items because it is the little things that bring to mind the biggest memories. When I was growing up, Sundays at our house consisted of going to church on Sunday morning, followed by a big Sunday dinner. Daddy loved fried chicken, and my mother made the best. Not only did she make good fried chicken, she also made the best gravy and mashed potatoes!

Going to church was always great fun because the entire family went to the same church—all my aunts, uncles and cousins, and there were many of us. Daddy had four sisters and three living brothers, all married with children. Everyone always knew when the Williams family was in church because altogether there were about thirty of us.

After church, we would often go to Grandma's for a big carry-in dinner, and of course Daddy always wanted Mother to take fried chicken. Mother would fix a big iron kettle full of fried chicken, and usually she would make a cake as well. Those are the best memories, the ones of being together on a Sunday afternoon.

My memory of the gravy bowl is the best. It is a little gray bowl with blue flowers of some kind. It is unusual, and I have never seen another one around, but it is what held the chicken gravy. It wasn't the bowl itself or the gravy in it but the memories that it held for me. It was the special times when the family sat down together, the evening meals when Daddy came home from work.

I recall the conversations of what was happening at school or what happened at work or the big Sunday dinners with grandparents, aunts and uncles. We had great times laughing and the adults all talking. At that time,

> "Some items you just can't part with."

children sat at the kids' table, and children didn't interrupt adult conversation. Parents didn't have to threaten for children to behave. Somehow, you just knew you better. Yes, those were special times of laughter and fun. My daughter was helping with the cleaning and organizing of the house for the auction that was fast approaching. She was like me, not wanting anything of great value. It was the simple items that held the most memories. In a drawer of an old antique sewing machine, she found the thimble that Daddy, her grandpa, used to hide somewhere in the room for the children to search for while waiting to open Christmas gifts.

We spent Christmas Eve at Mother's and Daddy's with cousins all there together. They were all so young, just little ones so excited about being together and Santa coming. Grandpa was in charge of entertaining the little ones, which of course wound them up even more. He loved Christmas, with the tree lights and the gathering of all the little ones he loved so. He would sneak off and ring the sleigh bells and holler, "Santa is flying over! You better be good!"

The children would run, jump and squeal with laughter. What fun! Daddy loved seeing the sparkle in their eyes while waiting for Santa. He would pass out candy and build with sugar the anticipation of the gifts that awaited them. Wonderful memories!

My son was the same with his choice of a keepsake. Again, it was of no real value. It was the green punch bowl that Grandma made the Christmas punch in. He loved her punch, and every year he now makes it for his family in that same bowl.

My daughter and son had great interest in the old pictures. They loved the pictures of their Grandma and Grandpa when they were young, like themselves—young and raising a family. Grandpa had hair, and Grandma looked like a movie star. Finding pictures of their mother as a baby or Uncle Jim's senior picture were a thrill to them. Life in a box—all the small little simple things that have the most memories.

CHAPTER 24

Family of the Heart

It seems as though AD hunted down our family and intended to destroy the very fabric of our family makeup. Daddy's mother, my grandma, showed signs of AD at a young age while in her early forties. As she aged, it became worse and worse. She started repeating herself and constantly worried about anything and everything.

I remember her being terrified of storms. She was so terrified that if it was a rainy day out, gray with no sun and it looked like rain, she wanted to head down to the cellar to take cover. If there was lightning and thunder, you might as well forget it. She wasn't coming out of the cellar until it had passed. Tornado warnings would come on TV and you might as well head to the cellar because she wouldn't have it any other way. She was terrified and would worry until Grandpa would open the door to the cellar.

> "The Christian heart is in every one of those brothers and sisters."

One has to ask, was that the early onset of AD? Were those truly early signs? However, everyone accepted that it was just Grandma, and life went on.

Through the years, my grandparents had hardships like all families. They married young and had nine children. Life was tough through the Great Depression, but they seemed to be tougher. Their third baby died at eighteen months from pneumonia. Grandma was heartsick, blaming herself, thinking the bottle she fed the baby was out of temperature and that was the cause of the baby's death.

Their fourth son died at age eighteen when he worked for the highway department. He was on break at lunchtime and fell asleep under the big water truck. When the lunchtime break was over and the whistle was blown, he never woke up, and the truck ran over him.

Grandpa was a fair Christian man. The county highway department wanted to charge the truck driver with neglect, but Grandpa went to court and would not press charges. He didn't believe the man was responsible for his son's death. It was an unfortunate accident.

Grandma never was the same and was always fretting about one thing and another. Son number one was sixty-eight when he died of brain cancer. He served in WWII and made it through the war but lost his battle to cancer. Grandma and Grandpa both felt it was just wrong to bury your children before yourselves.

The Christian heart is in every one of those brothers and sisters. They set an example of love that speaks highly of their parents. They have set the bar high when it comes to being a caregiver.

At the time of Grandma's illness and her diagnosis of AD, every one of the seven children that remained living were her caregivers. They took turns staying the night, cooking, cleaning and bathing her. She was taken care of in her home until her death. This set the example to be followed by the younger generation.

All the aunts were special in their own way. Aunt Sissy was taller than the rest of the Williams sisters, shapely and a knockout even in her eighties. She loved the Lord, and she told you about Him every time you would see her. She had five boys and always wanted a girl, but that was not to be. She always told me if she had had a girl, she would love one just like me.

Just the way she said your name, you knew she loved you. AD has her now, and my heart breaks every time I'm around her. She is taken care of by her boys, and again the youngest has the load, not that anyone is purposely doing that, but it is just how life goes. All the boys live miles away, and the one that chose to stay has the chores to do. I'm sure he would not have it any other way. I'm sure heartache is on the way, for he looks just like his father. I'm sure he will be mistaken for him many times before she processes out of this life.

Aunt Helen, Daddy's sister number three, has AD. She is the mother of my two cousins Sherra and John. Those two were my buddies growing up. Sherra, Miss Independent, was like my little sister. She was amazing, and we always loved to be together. We would laugh and giggle. Growing up, we shared a lot about dating boys, makeup, horses, books and movies.

John was a guy, but we had lots of crazy good times together as kids. Both are super intelligent. I'm not sure where all of Sherra's degrees are from, but she was a nurse on the heart team at the hospital for twenty years, then started teaching nursing at the local college. John graduated from Purdue and has been a surgical tech for the past twenty years.

It is now John and me. Sherra passed in the spring from a long fight with cancer. She came to the nursing home to check on me the day Daddy passed, and she also was giving me a heads-up that her recent doctor's appointment had shown a lump. She felt positive about it because she had gastric bypass surgery months earlier. When she had that done and with the weight loss, she felt like that was good they found the lump. She thought maybe without the weight loss, it would have gone undiscovered.

The cancer she had was the worst kind, and it was aggressive. My heart broke again as I lost my cousin, my little sister, my friend. John and I had a rough time, but I felt like it was more important for him to vent.

His father, Uncle Marvin, pretty much died in his arms a few years ago. Aunt Helen, John's mother, doesn't remember who he is, and now his sister Sherra is gone. Life is unfair at times, but we both understand how important it is to hang on to each other and ride this life out together. There is the special one, Aunt Mary, the youngest of the nine. My heart and her heart are bonded as she watched her parents go before her, as well as three of her brothers and two of her sisters diagnosed with AD. Her only son was killed in a car accident in his twenties. This woman is unbelievable, with a smile on her face showing the strength within her. She has climbed many mountains in her life and still is, but there is no question that God is her Savior.

CHAPTER 25

Some Days, Holidays and Precious Memories

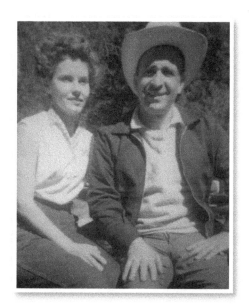

Some days, I wish my parents were with us again so I could hear the war stories one more time or just be with them before the illness. I wish for our silly talks, our conversations about nothing. We solved world problems many times over in our talks. I think of all the bantering back and forth while playing cards. Euchre is a Midwest card game, and my Daddy could play that game like no other! He was good and hard to beat!

They were always there. I could always count on them no matter what. They were always ready to listen, not always with answers, but they would be there to support me any way they could. I just miss them so much.

Daddy's energy and smile were priceless. Mother's calmness was so soothing. She never got too worked up about anything. She had a saying that she used many times in a caring voice: "Well, hmm, that's too bad."

She would remain very calm. She wasn't going to get upset about the situation you or anyone else were in. She didn't know what to do, so she wasn't going to get upset, nor was she going to jump in and try to do anything. It would work itself out!

After all these years, I now realize and understand more and more of why she said that phrase. Everyone has problems and situations to work out, and it is theirs to do so. She had the attitude that she had her own problems to take care of, and at times that was more than enough.

As I ponder the day, it is Thanksgiving. Thanksgiving is my holiday. I love to cook and fuss over my family, with all the eating, the closeness and the talking. I do and have always loved this holiday. It was always special to me to have Mother and Daddy come to our home for that day. In the early years, it involved early morning hunting then eating. We usually had the Macy's parade on TV and then the football games. There would be short naps and, of course, card playing. What a great time!

Mother and Daddy always loved coming. Mother especially enjoyed it because she didn't have to do the work. She always brought the cranberry salad and slaw, and even the kids loved Grandma's salad items.

One time. when they were shopping at a local department store, Daddy came across a pie holder. It was in the shape of a ceramic pumpkin. Mother said he had to buy it because he had to give it to me. When Daddy gave that to me, he just laughed and said, "Now you know I'm going to look for a pie in that every time I come down!"

I have to say, I didn't disappoint him. Just about every time they came, he had a pie in it. He would lift the lid and say, "Gracie, just look at that pie!"

I remember the last Thanksgiving they were at our home. Our daughter Amanda stopped by and picked them up and brought them down. Daddy wasn't driving, and neither was Mother any longer. Caregivers had been hired, and we gave them the day off until evening.

I know Amanda was terribly upset about their car. It needed to be taken in for repair. It kept dying. When it would come to a stop, the engine would die. She was still upset by the time she got to our house, not only about the car but about the indifference she was seeing in her grandma about getting the car fixed.

Amanda explained to Grandma that the car dying at the wrong time could be detrimental to them, and she would let me know about it when she got to the house. Grandma couldn't understand what I was going to do about it. Amanda said, "I'm pretty sure Mom will call someone to fix it. That is what Mom does, Grandma. She takes care of your business."

With that said, Amanda told me it was a noticeably quiet ride the rest of the way. When they arrived, they seemed to be okay and ready to eat.

I took the big ceramic pie over to Daddy as soon as we got him to sit down at the table. I said, "Daddy, look what we have for you!"

I opened the pie holder, and he smiled really big and said, "Look, Gracie, pumpkin pie! Isn't that pretty?"

They both loved the food and some of the talk. They took a nap, and after that, Amanda and I decided that I would take them home in my car, and Amanda drove Mother and Daddy's car back to their house just to be safe.

That was the last time they spent the Thanksgiving holiday with us. How I miss them! There was always such laughter and talking, with many discussions about the world, World War II, Okinawa and landing Ernie Pyle there. (My father was with Ernie Pyle the day he was killed.) We talked about the old days, business, the kids, the grandkids, you name it, we probably talked about it.

My parents were such special people, my people. I truly do not feel we are without them now. I'm very thankful for the Thanksgiving holidays and those memories that I have. I cherish those memories. "Precious memories, how they linger! How they ever flood my soul." That songwriter had it right. Precious Father, loving Mother.

Today I still have my ceramic pie holder and Mother's china. I can still hear my daddy being excited about pie and Mother always calling when they got home and saying, "Everything was so nice. We had such a good time."

Not only on those special holidays but every day I'm thankful they were my parents. I'm very blessed each and every day that they were my people. My parents are the ones who made me who I am today.

CHAPTER 26

Fly Away

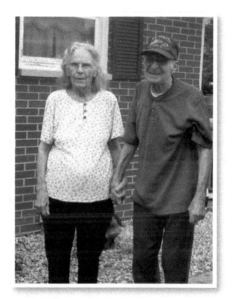

S ome bright morning when this life is over, I'll fly away.

We had Mother and Daddy's memorial service in November. Most of the preparations were complete. My brother came home after Daddy's passing and helped me with all the details earlier in the summer. We had ordered the headstone for the cremains, and it was ready to be placed upon their passing. The chapel was reserved, and a luncheon was planned in honor of our parents with many family and friends attending.

Our daughter Amanda gave a eulogy, and our son Blaine gave one as well. Both were very touching. You could hear in their voices how much their grandparents had been an example and in many ways an inspiration in their lives. As Amanda gave her eulogy, she touched on many things that were examples to her throughout her life. Let me share what she had to say that day.

Amanda's eulogy:

> I have started and stopped writing this many times over the last several weeks, wanting to say just the right words to honor these two people who I love, admire, respect and adore.
>
> I thought it best to tell you some things about them from my point of view as a granddaughter.
>
> I have felt lost many times since they have been gone, and I have come to realize that it is because I have lost my constants, my true north. I no longer have the comfort in the knowledge that no matter where on this planet I might be, the one thing that has never changed in my forty years is knowing that they are there, home on their beautiful farm.
>
> Then I realized that if I looked hard enough, there are things they taught me and memories I have of the way they lived their lives that will continue to be my guide in life. I could spend all day talking about these things, but here are a few of the most important lessons I learned from them.
>
> First: family is the most important thing. They each loved their parents, children, grand-children, great-grandchildren, brothers and sisters, and were proud of all of them. Grace kept every card each of you ever sent to her. She clipped and saved any newspaper articles that mentioned anyone she ever knew.

Second: work hard and be proud of what you have, but play hard too. They always made time for trips, long walks, fishing, and I am sure many of you have memories of buggy rides.

Third: believe it or not, Benny taught me that life is not fair. He never let me win, just because I was a kid, not at checkers or foot races, and I still say he cheated at euchre. He taught me that if you want to get ahead, you need to figure it out.

And last: get up early! I still struggle with this one. If you sleep in, you are missing out. When we were kids and stayed all night with them, Benny would stand outside the window or door and sound reveille until we would get up and have coffee and enjoy the sunrise with him before he started his day. He knew life was short and wanted to cram as much living into each day as possible.

All of these lessons, I will forever hold dear to my heart.

While cleaning out their house, I came across a book of poetry that Grandma and I had read from together often. The bookmark had slipped out and been picked up and put back in. I just knew it would not be in the same place she had left it, and I was upset that I would not know what she had been thinking about the last time she had the book open.

A few weeks later, I was having a rough day, and I was really crying over losing them both, wishing I could hold her hand one more time. I sat down on the floor and opened the book. I found so many pages marked with paper, all significant to the way I was feeling right then.

I would like to share two of them with you now.
Beautiful Hands
Such beautiful, beautiful hands,
They're neither white nor small;
And you, I know, would scarcely think
That they were fair at all.
I've looked on hands whose form and hue
A sculptor's dream might be,
Yet are these aged wrinkled hands
Most beautiful to me.
Such beautiful, beautiful hands!
Though heart were weary and sad
These patient hands kept toiling on
That the children might be glad.
I almost weep when looking back
To childhood's distant day!
I think how these hands rested not
When mine were at their play.
Such beautiful, beautiful hands!
They're growing feeble now,
And time and pain have left their mark
On hand and heart and brow.
Alas! alas! The nearing time—
And the sad, sad day to me,
When 'neath the daisies, out of sight,
These hands must folded be.
But, oh! beyond the shadowy lands,
Where all is bright and fair,
I know full well these dear old hands
Will palms of victory bear.
By Ellen M. H. Gates from the book *Heart Throbs*

Good-Bye

There is a word, of grief the sounding token;
There is a word bejeweled with bright tears,
The saddest word fond lips have ever spoken;
A little word that breaks the chain of years;
Its utterance must ever bring emotion,
The memories it crystals cannot die,
Tis known in every land, on every ocean—
Tis called "Good-Bye."

Said to have been written by Ah Foo Lin, a Chinese student in a friend's album from the book *Heart Throbs*

In the weeks since they have been gone, I have shed many a tear, but I have also smiled through some of those tears, remembering some of the best times I shared with the two most beautiful souls I have ever known.

These things will always remind me of them and cause me to smile or shed a tear:

- long gravel driveways and hickory nuts
- sleigh bells and saddle leather
- warm fresh watermelon with salt
- the smell of cedar
- basketball and popcorn
- bread and butter
- tree swings
- Easter eggs and checkerboards
- fishing poles and books of poems
- sunrise and beautiful sunsets
- horseshoes and butterflies
- boat anchors and daisies

Thank you, Amanda!

What was so amazing was our son Blaine was stationed in Okinawa at the time, and he and Amanda had very little time to talk. They had not put their thoughts together about their eulogies. However, they both had a lot of the same thoughts and life lessons to share. Both eulogies were very touching.

There were a few funny stories told about both Mother and Daddy, and a lot of tears flowed that day. My uncle Kenny is a minister and has always been a joker of sorts. Of course, he had several funny stories to tell about Mother and Daddy, and there were a few we knew nothing about.

One comes to mind about how they had all been at my grandparents' home one evening, and Uncle Kenny had just bought a new Honda motorcycle. Mother thought that it looked like so much fun that she got on it, and Uncle Kenny took her for a ride, to everyone's surprise. She went on and on about how much fun that was. Now my parents enjoyed their buggy rides so much, so Mother told Uncle Kenny, "My ride doesn't go as fast as yours!"

He went on to tell about the nine bushels of morel mushrooms Daddy found one time. There were lots of stories over a long life shared by both.

Oddly, there have been several people named Williams who have been part of this story. There is one I especially will always hold dear to my heart: the lovely hospice minister, Allissa Williams. She came to the nursing home and helped sing my daddy to heaven. She has a beautiful voice! She graced us with her voice again at the service. I'm sure it is a heavenly voice, one the angels hear.

Veterans gave their salute, with the firing of the twenty-one guns to Dad. I was handed the flag for his service. It brings you back to reality—the hard reality—that Dad and Mom are gone, and they are not ever going to come back. There are so many memories they left to all of us.

As we left the chapel, balloons were released. We had bought balloons for the great-grandchildren to release in Mother and Daddy's honor. I remember that I walked toward their headstone and looked up as my grandchildren released balloons, and I whispered, "Fly high, Daddy and Mother. Fly high!"

As I looked up in a tree, there was a balloon hung up in the branches. It was just hanging there, and as I watched, the most amazing thing happened. Another balloon went past, as if to help the one that was hung up to release, and they went flying off together! No other balloons were around; all had drifted out of sight except those two.

How sweet the sight, the symbolism of togetherness! The one waited for the other; one was in trouble and the other came to the rescue. Mother and Daddy were married for sixty-eight years, and I know they were very close and very admiring of each other. They always had respect for one another. When one was in trouble or upset, the other one was always there—through thick and thin and in sickness and health. They were there for each other.

My father was an old-school, "hold the door open for a lady" type man. I have no doubt in my mind that he held the door open for Mother when she arrived in heaven, his beautiful Gracie. He would never leave her behind, and he didn't that day as they flew high together.

ABOUT THE AUTHOR

Teresa Williams Trotter has been a Christian since the age of twenty and has been active in every church she has attended throughout her life. She has been a successful businesswoman, having owned a cookie store in a mall, a cake-decorating business and an ice cream / lunch drive-in. She and her husband, Joe, owned a highly successful sporting goods store until their retirement.

Teresa and Joe were very instrumental in developing a rehab house called the Luke House for drug addiction. They spent a few years renovating an old house and served on the board to ensure that the Luke House would open. Their thoughts and hopes were that if it helped one life to change, then the endeavor was worth every minute of time.

Teresa and Joe have five children between them, twelve grand-children and one great-grandchild. They also are owned by an extremely spoiled Yorkshire terrier named Rex.

Teresa and Joe are both avid fishermen and hunters and enjoy camping, boating and geocaching. They love family and friends, gatherings and celebrations. They are also ardent card players and are hard to beat! Their motto is "Life is good, and God is great!"

Teresa is available for book signings and to speak to groups. You may also request a personalized bookplate for yourself or for gift copies. Please contact Teresa at Psalm46.10Teresa@gmail.com.

CPSIA information can be obtained
at www.ICGtesting.com
Printed in the USA
BVHW092356150421
605036BV00010B/1511